W9-BXY-630

Who Do I Become When I Am No Longer Me?

Stories of Illness, Injury, Chronic Pain, Aging and Dying

Susanne Carlson

VANTAGE PRESS
New York

FIRST EDITION

All rights reserved, including the right of
reproduction in whole or in part in any form.

Copyright © 2003 by Susanne Carlson

Published by Vantage Press, Inc.
516 West 34th Street, New York, New York 10001

Manufactured in the United States of America
ISBN: 0-533-14344-6

Library of Congress Catalog Card No.: 2002106738

0 9 8 7 6 5 4 3 2 1

Contents

Acknowledgments

To my mentor, Ashley Montagu, Ph.D. I only wish he had lived long enough to see the published fruition of his years of dedication to my thinking and learning process. No one in my educational realm, from kindergarten through graduate school, did more to stimulate me, challenge me, require me to come to my senses, to embrace my own knowing, and look carefully at all that was in my environment. A gifted and witty teacher, educator, philosopher, social anthropologist, Dr. Montagu required me to view all that I knew in one sense, or field, to find a point of integration in all of the others. He broadened my perspective to all that is related. He required that I find the symmetry in all that is human and humane. He would not settle for my limited, constricted vision of one system. If a process existed in human physiology as a system, then he required that I find a similar model in sociology or anthropology or anatomy. It is through the realization of these patterns in process that I began to observe differently the world around me. I am forever in his debt.

To Nancy Ryles. It was she who named this book and demanded that I write it. It is Nancy, her husband, Vern, and her other immediate and extended family members who reminded me daily that I knew something about living and dying and that it needed to be shared. I thank them deeply for their sustained support.

To the many patients that make up the stories I am about to tell. Twenty-five years is a long time to practice anything. One would think, after twenty-five years, you would be accomplished at something. Medicine isn't like that. I am every bit as much a

v

beginner after twenty-five years as I was when I started. I do trust myself a bit more. I know to respect my clinical judgment, but that's about all. Medicine changes so quickly, and patients present new problems so diligently, that to become a master of any form of medicine is an illusion at best. I love that we call our setting "a practice," and that we call those we see "patients." *Patience* is what they need to stand by us as we attempt to practice the balance of art and science.

These stories are of patients I have seen over my quarter of a century as a practitioner. I have changed their names and enough of the details to protect their privacy. In some instances, I have blended several patients into one story, as if they were one. Perhaps they had the same disease or have similar stories. Some of these patients are alive. Others have died. In any case, they are all alive in my memory. Their stories remain a part of the depth of my soul. The intimacy and dedication to growth each demonstrated is nothing short of heroic.

As we embrace a new millennium, I am stunned by the number of people who talk and write about the lack of heroes, courage, or discipline that is displayed in our society. I am saddened, as there are multitudes who walk among us who could and would serve as heroes if we only noticed . . . stories that would fill our hearts with courage and, most importantly for us, hope. Attitudes that, on a daily basis, show not only discipline, but stamina.

To my children, born or acquired, that I count among my best advisors, my source of humor, my sense of humility and humanity. They have each endured me, humored me, and brought me to my senses. They stimulated my creativity, corrected my facts, and altered my perspective. I am forever in their debt.

To my guardian angels: David Pool, the friend who gave me full support and great critique of my writing, Adrinne Kieth, Susan Hansen and Mary Fellows who served as editors, and to all of the doctors at Kaiser Permanente Oregon, and Oregon Health

Sciences University, who tolerated my educating them, who further educated me, and who provided the medical care and human touches I needed to learn about and feel my changes due to multiple sclerosis.

Who Do I Become When I Am No Longer Me?

Nancy

Nancy lay on one couch, coffee cup in hand, sun streaming through the windows behind her. I lay on the couch opposite her with my own coffee cup, my feet propped on the arm rest. Her husband, Vern, sat in a chair between us. It seemed like a normal Sunday morning with newspapers strewn on the coffee table. We could have been best of friends sharing a quiet Sunday conversation. We were friends, that part was true. We were launched, however, on a path that would make us more than friends, and explore forms of intimacy none of us could have imagined.

Nancy had just returned from what was to be a family trip to California to babysit her firstborn grandson. It had become, one seizure, a hospital stay, and diagnostic hell later, the beginning of the end. Nancy had an inoperable brain tumor.

I had first met Nancy in the world of politics, children's politics, public activism politics, state politics. Nancy was busy. She was an under-employed woman with a flair for the challenge of life and a drive like a Porsche. She was smart, cute, and full of "vim and vigor." She was my kind of woman. She wore her passion on her sleeve and in her heart. She was direct and honest. She had one of the driest, sharpest wits that I had ever heard. She was quick with a response that would be simultaneously filled with fact and humor. She ate junk food, Twinkies were her favorite, when there was no time to eat. She ran instead of walked, and spoke faster than most people could listen. She was respected. No matter where her position fell in relationship to an issue, everyone could count on her to listen, consider, change her mind if it made sense to her to do so, or challenge your thinking with facts and arguments that would penetrate your resolve. She was everything anyone in public would want of a school board member, a state legislator, a committee chairperson, an advisory council member, or a think-tank policy setter. She was great!

It was perfect that it was Nancy who conceived the idea for this book and named it. That morning, we lay considering her options, talking over her medical advance directive and outlining possible steps and adaptations that would need to be made. Most of us would be deep in our narcissistic self-absorption. We would lie in our self-pity and inner bartering to stave off the ultimate death. Nancy, on the other hand, suggested that I write a book about pain, trauma, aging, and dying. A book about stories. A book that would allow other families to talk about the complexity of life's changes. Nancy's question to me, "Sue, who do I become when I am no longer me?" summed the context of the book up in one sentence.

Who do any of us become when we are no longer ourselves? Who are we in the phase of life when we are "disintegrating" instead of integrating? How do we explain ourselves *to* ourselves or others when we can no longer find ourselves among the remnants of what we were? Where do we find the words for the explanation of *how* we have changed, or *what* we have changed into? Who are we when we cannot see, hear, smell, taste, or feel? How do we describe our experience when we can no longer speak or write or cry? How do we hold an image of ourselves when we can no longer hold ourselves, when we can no longer move or walk, turn or sit by ourselves? How do we gather ourselves when we cannot get to the bathroom at all, no less in "time"? Who are we when the body that we've known and depended upon lapses, won't cooperate, won't "shut up" long enough for us to sleep?

2

I know these questions deeply myself now as I struggle with multiple sclerosis. Having lost and regained my vision, I am acutely aware of my need to see as much as I can in every moment. I never know when my neurology and my sight will lapse again, perhaps never to return. At least each time I look and see I can commit the sights, patterns, colors, landscapes, and forms to memory. I can soothe myself saying, *At least I will have the memory of this moment.* I am even more afraid of losing the memory.

Who do I become when I am no longer me? Who am I as I become a different form of me? How do I both assure others in my life that I am becoming a new me and am not leaving them yet, all the while reminding them and myself, that I am not capable of being the old me? How do I remain in my senses as my senses change from day to day? How do I trust myself when my self is altering, or is altered by medications, on a daily basis? How do I learn to make sense of my self-worth and self-image when they both change every time I look in the mirror or review my thinking, (that presumes I still can review my thinking). If the people in my life liked me when they choose to be with me, do they continue to like me when I am not like myself? Can they still like me when I don't even *like* myself anymore?

I know these are the real questions. I've heard them countless times. I've considered them over and over. We don't talk about these things openly in this society. We don't consider these topics coffee conversations or dinner table discussions. We don't have maps that direct us past the obstacles that these questions raise. We press the issues away. We deny or rationalize them. We justify away our need to deal with them. We hold our independence with such ruthlessness that we hold others far away. Yet, these are such valuable lessons.

We could teach all those around us if we could hold our internal fears and self-talk conversations externally. This society does not make room for the weak or ailing. We can see that in the difficulty we have had in producing laws for the disabled, no less following them with pride and diligence. Unfortunately, that leaves those in pain, in disability, in disease, in aging, and in dying doing so quietly.

Isolation is a source of deprivation for an entire civilization. If we don't appreciate dying, how can we possibly appreciate living? If we can't honor our disability, how do we truly acknowledge our ability? If we cannot feel our disease, how do we embrace our ease, our wellness? If we are not willing to touch the possibility of becoming injured, ill, disabled, aged, or dead, then how do we rehearse these events so that we are prepared to deal with them physically, emotionally, mentally, and spiritually, when they occur? They *will* occur. They will occur to each and every one of us.

We rehearse. We rehearse our lives constantly, in our waking and sleeping states. We rehearse events, decisions, discussions, and postures. We rehearse so that we can be prepared. The more we rehearse, the better our presentation of self. Children do this with such ease, I often wish we could, as adults, embrace this ability once again. Children set neurological pathways with repetitious movement. They learn to speak, walk, talk, eat and sleep with rehearsal. We, as a species, are repetitious learners. The more we do something, the more efficient the activity becomes. Some are more disciplined in their rehearsing, others of us do much of it unconsciously. But we rehearse, nevertheless.

There are no pat answers. There are no fine lines on maps. There are no perfect ways. There are no right or wrong responses. There are only stories. People doing the very best they can with the skills, knowledge, and experiences they have accumulated in their lives, to deal with change.

At no time in civilization have so many lived so long and so well, that we can die of degeneration. At no time in history have we had the technology to diagnose so early in a disease process. We are able to know, understand, and be watchful of ourselves as we move

4

through the changes associated with illness, injury, pain, pain management, aging and dying. We are the pioneers.

I have long loved the Chinese folktale of the farmer in a small, isolated village in northern China. He was the richest man in the village because he owned a horse. One day the horse ran away. "Oh, the bad luck," said all the villagers. "Good luck, bad luck, who is to know?" responded the farmer. A year or so went by, and one day, the horse returned. In the interim of time, the horse had foaled. The farmer was instantly twice as rich as he now had two horses. "Oh, the good luck," responded the villagers. "Good luck, bad luck, who is to know?" stated the farmer. Months later, the farmer's oldest son was green-breaking the foal when he was thrown off the young horse, severely breaking his leg. "Oh, the bad luck," cried the villagers. "Good luck, bad luck, who is to know?" replied the farmer. Two weeks later, the Chinese army came through the village and constricted all of the able-bodied young men, except for the farmer's son. After all, what good is a soldier with a broken leg? "Oh, the good luck!" exclaimed the villagers. "Good luck, bad luck, who is to know?" sighed the farmer. This story has no ending. I heard it told in China where every Chinese person on the bus had to add another chapter. They all told me it was the story of China and the perseverance of the Chinese people. It was with much honestly and laughter as each extension of the tale was told.

The Chinese love luck. Luck, for them, is a very valuable commodity. I have never identified with luck as the Chinese do. I often wish I could. I alter the context of this story slightly in my response. I, when taking the part of the farmer, respond with "Good news, bad news, who is to know?" I understand the concept of "news" better than I understand the concept of "luck." Every patient has heard me say it. Each time I say it, it reminds me to follow the concept. *Hold your judgment, you just never know what will happen next!*

Pain, trauma, disease, aging, and dying are like this. Hold your judgment, you never know what will happen next, or how it will turn out. We can never know how we will adapt. We watch others adapt. We often do not watch closely enough to celebrate with them, witness the changes and adaptation for them, or grieve the losses with them. We are not taught, in society, to appreciate the changes of seasons. The dance of the Earth in her day-to-day changes. Some of those changes known as storms, we often call calamities. We forget that we adapt to the Earth's changes daily. The angle of the sun, the clouds overhead, the force of the wind require changes in each of us physically, mentally, emotionally. We are animals, too. We are connected to this Earth.

We attempt to hold ourselves away from these forces that require adaptation by pretending they have little or no effect upon us. We live in our environmentally controlled houses, communicate far beyond the extent of our voice, and travel faster than our feet can carry us in a day. We hold fast to our belief that we, as humans, are above the forces of nature and the forces of the Earth. Adapters that we are, we have adapted in ways that tease us into the belief that no further adaption is required. Our final adaptation often comes in our dying. In some of us, it comes before death when we are forced to adapt because of pain, injury, or disease. When we are forced to realize that as good as we are, as capable as we've become in our technological advancements, as resourceful we are with our money-purchased things, we must still adapt to pain, illness, trauma and the changes they demand in our bodies, in ourselves.

The Gift of Time

Max

I received a phone call from a colleague who worked for a large local health maintenance organization. She was referring a patient to me. She informed me at the beginning of the conversation that this man had AIDS and asked if I was willing to see him. This was early in the AIDS saga; the stage when we in society and medicine were all mildly hysterical about the "new plague" of Acquired Immune Deficiency Syndrome; the disease carried with it all of the social stigmas of how it had been "acquired."

Max was in pain. He had relentless edema (swelling). He was trying to continue to work, but his pain and stiffness made it nearly impossible. My colleague thought I could help him. Actually, it was more loaded than that. She said, "Nothing else is working. He's desperate and I don't know of anyone else who will see him." His HMO insurance coverage would not pay for my work. This patient not only had to make a giant leap of faith, but a huge pocketbook leap along with it.

I love medical history, almost as much as I love medicine, physiology, pathophysiology, and anatomy. I love bodies. I love complexity. I love the miracle of wellness, illness, and healing. I love the change and growth that drive our understanding of these subjects. Nothing in medicine is ever boring.

Actually, I have never seen the same body twice. I have seen people weekly for months and years on end, but the human body changes at a cellular level, and at a tissue level many times over as these time periods go by. Some aspect of the person remains, usually their experiences, memories, history . . . the "brain" stuff of their self. Their body changes within a week. My job, in many cases, is to be the "witness" of these profound changes. Body changes happen as a nuance. We, the person inhabiting the body, seldom notice these small changes. It isn't until the change is large enough that it causes pain, illness, or alteration in function that we bring these changes to a level of consciousness.

I have spent much commuter time contemplating my "job" as a facilitator and educator to the process of health, life, and death. I have pondered the boundaries of saying "no" or "I can't" countless times. I am frankly not very good at either.

Why wouldn't I see him? How could I turn down someone who had fallen into the limbo land of medicine? As great as modern medicine is, it isn't perfect. Far from it. We do have wonder drugs. We just don't have wonder drugs for everything that humans need for repair or pain. We do have wonder surgeries. We just can't do surgery on everything that can go wrong. We do have spectacular technology for diagnosis. It's just that often we end up knowing too much with no way to deal with the information. It's a truly "good news, bad news" situation.

Max arrived at my office at the crack of dawn a week later. My office hours begin at 7:00 AM to facilitate the working multitudes. Max was a medical professional himself. A pathologist by training, he ran a large medical laboratory. He had no idea how he had gotten AIDS. His one sexual partner showed no demonstration of the disease.

Max was suffering not only from a fatal disease but the social stigmas surrounding that disease. Once his diagnosis had been made, it was presumed that he was a homosexual. This extremely quiet, reserved male human being felt violated at every level. Had he been diagnosed with cancer, the process and outcome would not have looked much different, but the empathy levels and privacy issues would have been much less malevolent.

Max certainly could have contracted the disease "on the job," where he dealt with human excretions daily. Evidently, that thought had not occurred to anyone. I found this obvious possibility a cosmic giggle. Each of the professionals in his lab were as vulnerable as he was. Each of us in the medical profession were as vulnerable as he was. Any of *us* could also contract this disease as a consequence of exposure on the job. This is, in fact, what drives the hysteria and the stigma. We want to push our own vulnerability back. In order to accomplish that, we must make generalities about others and somehow separate "them" from "us." We must name and blame, and in this case, shame the person away from us. We must make him, name him as different . . . a homosexual, to give us an illusion of control. This separation allows us to, at least intellectually, define our control. He *has* to be different somehow from us or we, too, could fall victim to a deadly disease. The obvious logical sequence would have to have been: If you are in medicine, and could contract AIDS, therefore you must be a homosexual male. As humans, we are slightly one bead off center when it comes to logic.

Max lived alone. Married to his work, he had chosen to enjoy his nieces and nephews as his "children" and a weekend companion of long-standing instead of a constant partner. He was very shy. The thought of being massaged, having appendages moved out of his control, and having tensions explored that he wasn't even aware of was a huge shift in his consciousness. He didn't know how to let go of control. He spoke about his control over his lab, the protocols, the processes, the standards of practice, his house, his dress, and his appearance with great honor and pride. We had to work together weekly on his learning to let go of the control of his body so that I could move it, massage it, and manage it for his comfort. It was a process!

The therapy also gave him pain relief. His pain medications dropped and his functioning at work went back up. His improvement was short-lived. At the suggestion of an attorney friend of his, he had filed a worker's compensation claim for his illness. No one in the state had ever filed a claim suggesting they had contracted AIDS in the line of duty. *What a concept!* This was during a time when blood samples and other human fluids were manipulated using pipettes. Many lab processes were done "by hand," with hands unprotected. As a result, the lab administration went ballistic. They attempted to prove his illness was not work-related, but rather was a result of homosexuality. They began a long process of discrediting his work. They publicly announced and denounced their perceived betrayal of his workplace due to his claim. His coworkers joined the fray. Perhaps they were not wanting to acknowledge their own vulnerability to a disease process possible in the workplace. All in all, the stress on Max was obvious.

If I had ever wondered about stress hormones and their effect on the body, I was able to bear witness as an immediate observer. If I had ever wanted to see the rage and range of stress hormones on an already compromised physiological system, I had an available textbook, lying on a treatment table weekly, before my eyes. His skin broke down. His hair fell out. His eyes swelled and crusted. His luster faded. His very life blood was taken away.

I watched a body process that I could describe in medical terms. The translation was much harder and much sadder in our commonly used words. Was Max dying from a disease or was Max dying from a disease that we, society, were thrusting upon him? Was Max dying because of *society's* pressures and emotional abuses?

I adore words. The roots of words are like a history lesson through time for me. *Integrare*, is Latin, meaning whole. *Integer*, a whole number. *Integrated*, a whole system that is congruent. *Integument*, the skin, the whole covering of the human body, and the largest organ of the body. Skin is amazing. It can take over where other organs either leave off or can't fully accomplish their jobs.

I have my favorite bone, the scapula. The pelvis is a close second. I love the contours, the ridges, the soft lines, the brute strength. I have my favorite muscle, the quadratus lumborum. It has a variety of attachments and movements. It has skill as a prime mover and as a stabilizer. It has ability to respond in microscopic movements to correct the very nuance of posture; its diligence in supporting a baby, providing the "hip seat," even at the expense of its own fatigue. I have my favorite organs, the liver and the skin. I cannot ever choose between them. I list them first and second, alternating their rankings, but I cannot eliminate one of them and place it a true second. I love these organs because of their complexity, and their myriad functions. I love the effect they have on the entire body. I love their subtlety. I love their disasters. I love that they recreate themselves. I love their ability to repair.

There are not many people who have a favorite bone, muscle, or organs. It is too bad. I truly believe that if we deeply understood how wondrous this human body is, we would all treat it quite differently.

Max loved pathology. We built a great deal of our mutual trust around our passionate and animated conversations about physiology and pathophysiology. Our weekly hour together would go by with my hands, thankfully, disconnected from my brain, working away at one process while we discussed blood, urine, slides, and disease.

As the stress Max experienced wore through to his soul, he found himself giving up the fight. He agreed to resign, short of being fired. He agreed to accept his retirement, short of fully vested. He agreed that his disease was, in fact, in the way of his work. By the time everyone and everything had hammered at him, he was too ill to continue in his work. He lost control of that which had been his true reason for living—the work that he had devoted his entire life to accomplishing, the piece of significance in his life where he honored and produced for the society.

We all know stories about the person who plans on traveling, gardening, reading, visiting friends upon retirement, but who dies the day after doing so. Have we pondered the person who fully expected to die before retiring, who planned on coping with his dying by working?

Max went home.

Max was much too sick now to come into the clinic. I couldn't say no when he asked if I would come to his home once a week. Max lived in a beautifully furnished cottage. When I fantasize about cottages, my mind goes to *Snow White and the Seven Dwarfs* . . . a rolling roof bungalow with windows and window boxes, and winding paths by fancy flowers and bird baths. His house wasn't far from my fantasies. It was quite a study in stunning beauty and small, detailed features. Max's cottage fit all of my fantasies perfectly. He had obviously spent years developing the gardens, with nooks and crannies that made up a world away from the world. Paths that wandered back upon themselves in such a way that following them allowed you to feel like you'd taken a long stroll. Birds called to the blends of food and nurture. Colors and blends of colors that illuminated Max's artistry. The same complexities that he loved in medicine were translated over and over in his choice of plants, textures of path covering, sculptures, bird baths, water flowing, and color. Max was also a gardener.

As wonderful as the cottage and garden were while he was well, they were awful with him ill. The problems were notable immediately. There were stairs everywhere. Two steps down to the kitchen, three steps up to the living room, two corners and three steps into the sun room. Seven steps and one sharp corner to an upstairs bedroom and bath. Nine steps, two landings and one corner into a downstairs bedroom, bathroom, and laundry room. There were oriental throw rugs. Artifacts and fancy furniture everywhere—gorgeous, uncomfortable furniture. The kitchen was built for dwarfs, not wheelchairs.

I could not imagine how we were going to make this all work for him. Yet, he was adamant. He was going to stay home. He had lost control over most of his life, he wasn't about to lose this, too. The house, however, was a nursing nightmare.

There were a few inexpensive things that could be done. A gas log was plumbed into his bedroom fireplace so that he wouldn't have to carry firewood downstairs to enjoy the fires that he loved so much. Oriental scatter rugs were replaced with room-sized oriental rugs that would be anchored by the heavy furniture when his gait became shuffled. A truly compassionate oriental rug dealer in town traded and discounted to make the whole process work.

Max refused a hospital bed. It simply made him feel too sick. He was indeed so sick, that the thought of making him feel more sick sat like a plague of its own on my spirit. His parents arrived to care for him. They were in their seventies, and bending over a double bed, walking thousands of stairs, maneuvering medical equipment around doors and up and down stairs was as beastly for them as for him. Max's parents were wonderful, proud farmers from another state. They were foreigners to the city. Just shopping and running errands was a chore. Meeting three or four medical appointments a week outside the house was a disaster. It became apparent that we needed to call in the cavalry.

Friends familiar to the city were drummed up. They all responded with such enthusiasm that it took a computer to set forth a schedule so they only had to invest an hour or so every ten or eleven days in order to accomplish the multiple tasks.

I believe that when we are ever faced with the impending death of someone near to us, we need to give time. We simply should not wait until they are dead to send flowers and a note to their family. Give time. Do the *doing*. Give one hour, so that a primary-care giver can take a nap, take a walk, or soak in a bath. Time ahead of death is far kinder than flowers on a grave. Give one hour making food to bring in. Give time.

13

Max and his parents had to be lovingly shepherded through a huge transition of changing roles, rules, rituals and biological imperatives. We are not supposed to have our adult children precede us in death. It breaks down the natural order. Max had left the family farm for other work. No one in the family had understood. There were years of hard feelings that had to be worked through and very little time to work through them. There was grief. There was hardship. There were issues of who would be taking care of the parents. There were the surroundings that seemed to the parents like fluff. This was far from the familiar, practical furniture in the farmhouse. There were the stories of worldwide travels Max had taken. His parents had never cared to hear about these stories. Confronted with the pictures on the walls, these stories now needed to be told. They needed to expand their understanding of who Max was. It was all very confusing, as Max was, in his own perception, contracting from who he had been.

Surrounded by his friends and family, Max felt better. He could not make sense of the discrepancies between his perfectly manicured former home and the fact that there was a portable commode in the sun room. He could not fully justify the harsh reality that he was placed in the living room and had a two-room option for the entire day just because moving him up and down the stairs was too onerous a task for any of his caregivers. He was served his meals on a tray. He met his medical caregivers and held court in his previously seldom-used formal living room. For all of the difficulties, Max got to stay home. He held up under his own weight as much as he could bear. He moved himself around his house for as long as he could. His sense of humor blossomed. He could, and would, tease everyone about his bouts of stubbornness and his "smelly farts."

Max began to give away himself. He gave his lifetime of collected treasures to the people who were the real treasures of his life. He would tell the story that belonged to each item as he gave it away. In doing so, he shared a piece of himself. He was losing himself, and his belongings. Each friend went away with not only a treasure, but the treasured story that provided the context of how he had acquired it, or what part it played in his life. He and his belongings went on in everyone else's being.

Max did not die of AIDS. Max, like so many others, died of the opportunistic diseases a weakened immune system allows. Max had a stroke and was finally overcome by pneumonia.

On one of the final nights, two of his male friends had arrived to cook dinner. Neither of these men had ever been around anyone who was dying. When they had volunteered to help, they had both asked to be assigned tasks that could be completed far from the "scene." It took months before they could be talked into doing the cooking of a meal in the "dwarf kitchen," not because it was easy, (it wasn't) but because Max was hardly able to eat anything. His nose worked great though, so smelling the food being prepared and cooked was far more joy for him than the actual eating.

This night, the usual banter from the sun room wasn't there. There wasn't the usual "I smell the olive oil, it is too hot" (Max was a terrific cook himself) coming from the "couch seat chief." I arrived, greeted Max with a touch on his hand, and went to the kitchen door (there simply wasn't enough room for three of us to be in the kitchen at once) to find these two adult men crying their eyes out. It took several minutes of self-control and Kleenex before I could discern that they had come to the realization that Max would not be eating or smelling dinner that night. They were not going to have to prepare a tray to take to the living room. They would be sitting in the dining room, surrounded by elegance, eating dinner on Spode china by themselves. Death was real. Death was close. They were right there. Humanity had outlived fear.

Sight, Insight, "In-sight"
Sarah

Sarah was an airhead. She was a space cadet. She could be counted on to get nothing done. She lived in her own world. She had come to the clinic to "experience herself," whatever that meant. She was the epitome of the "new age energy spirit." She meditated, did yoga, didn't really work, lived on nothing at all, and, frankly floated through life. My only contact with her was in passing, usually as she floated by me coming into or going out of the clinic after a "massage experience."

I do clinical work, so my days are not filled with the floaters. Instead, they are made up of working on postsurgical adhesions or restricted movements. I spend my time retraining neurological patterns in stroke victims and Parkinsonian patients. I get the burn patients who need skin to be loosened, or the children with cerebral palsy who need to learn to turn over. Mine is the referral where the patient is a pedestrian hit by a car at twenty-five miles per hour, and has been surgically "fixed," but is still in pain, and whose physician is fearful of the pain medications and addiction. I get the pregnant moms who have so much ligament flaccidity that they don't have a leg to stand on. I am the recipient of the calcified tendinitis or the sprained ankle. I get to labor on the jaw that has been reconstructed, wired shut for eight weeks, and then doesn't move when the wires are cut. My days are never spent doing relaxation massage. I would not know how to do a relaxation massage. I would find a muscle that needs to be worked on and an hour would go by with the other 99 percent of the body untouched. I love clinical massage. I am well suited and trained for the work I do, but it is a "good news, bad news" experience because I simply can't do a full-body relaxation massage. It is too boring!

I was therefore shocked to find Sarah on my schedule. I was, frankly, terrified! I was angry at the front desk for making such a stupid error in scheduling, therefore keeping away someone who really needed my skills. It was not until my ranting and raving stopped for lack of breath, when the receptionist informed me that Sarah was medically referred and the referral letter was on my desk. *"Neck tension and headaches, please send me your findings and treatment plan,"* was the extent of the letter. I wondered how I could get her to actually lie on the table, as opposed to floating above it, and even pondered the old "nursing restraints" as I laughed at the image.

Sarah appeared several days later, her usual airhead self. I must admit that several "no brains, no headaches" jokes had rolled through my head. I wondered how someone who never entered the influence of gravity could possibly have tension, no less, enough tension to cause headaches. I am not proud of these prejudices or tacky unprofessional thoughts, but I am, in my humanity, subject to them, nevertheless. I am thankful, these many years later, that I never uttered these thoughts to her, or anyone else for that matter. The path this young woman of twenty-eight was about to embark upon was truly a path of heroic measure. I realize now that she may not ever have really been an airhead, but rather an angel sent to earth to teach us strength of character, dignity, and perseverance.

Sarah closed her eyes and entered a dream-like state that I had never seen. She was there in body, but not in consciousness. I gathered the usual data, pursued the usual medical questions, wrote my take on the presented history, and had to force every answer out of her. Every question I asked seemed to yank her back from a status of semi-consciousness. Finally, she informed me that she was simply not going to answer anymore of my questions, because opening her eyes gave her the headache I was supposed to "fix." I really hate it when this happens. I have learned over and over that the combination of ignorance and arrogance is lethal. I have been the perpetrator of both in my need for information upon which to make a decision for treatment. In that moment, I had to pursue one more question, although I did let her know it was fine to keep her eyes closed while answering. Eye contact is something we're trained to do in medicine. *Make that eye contact!* I did need to ask if she had told her doctor about the connection between her eyes being open and her headaches and neck tension. She informed me that he hadn't asked.

Medicine is complex. If we could sit in an audience and watch medicine as a play, we would be entertained by the humor of it all, the precariousness of the dancing between the patient and the practitioner, and the tragedy caused by miscommunication or misplaced context. Like watching a play, we can see a plot unfold, but are helpless to do anything about it. The frequency of clinical failure based on the practitioner not asking the right questions, or the patient not volunteering the necessary information, is absolutely astounding to me.

I worked on Sarah's neck. It was not a neck filled with tension. It was not a neck loaded with "hot spots." It was not made up of short, tight bands of muscles. My practice has always been to look for three findings that match the diagnosis. If I cannot find a correlation in actual physical findings to three pieces of data that I acquire, I back way off and begin the process again. I had looked for three physical findings on Sarah's neck to help verify or establish information toward a diagnosis. I had come up short. I could not establish an "ah-ha!"

Necks are amazing. If you want to fully appreciate what I am about to explore, put the book down and do this one little exercise. Place your thumbs touching together in front on your neck. Wrap your hands around your neck and find your index finger in back. If your fingers do not meet, feel around and try to establish how far apart your index fingers are from each other. Others of you may find that your index fingers do meet with a point to point touch. Still others of you may find that your index fingers overlap. Note where they touch each other. Now, away from your neck, replicate that hand position and look at the size of the hole your fingers describe. Look carefully at the circumference and the diameter. Now, if you will, imagine what is contained in that circle. There are twenty-six or so muscles. There is a bony vertebral column containing a spinal cord. There are four primary blood vessels, each about the size of your own thumb. Our own body is accurately proportioned, with numerous smaller blood-carrying vessels. There are primary and secondary nerves. There is an esophagus and a trachea. All of that, and a job to do, besides. The need to balance our eleven to fifteen pounds of head on our body. We treat our necks with indifference. We subject the neck, not only to wear and tear, but to brutal attack in the form of sports activities and head positions. It is truly a miracle that this primary conduit of life itself is as vulnerable as it is, and somehow manages to survive us!

I spent an hour on Sarah's neck. Her neck and I became good friends. I memorized the contours and crevasses of each muscle. I felt pulses and found the string-like contours of nerves. I studied the range of motion. I had a great time exploring it all, but, as I stated in my report back to the doctor, there was no tension to speak of. In fact, if anything, there was too little tension. Hyper-mobile is the clinical word we use to define too much range of motion, in any direction, at any particular joint. Every other joint I explored in her body was the same, hyper-mobile. Could her hyper-mobility be why she appeared to float? Might the precariousness of her balancing act with loose, hyper-mobile joints be causing her headaches? What was the relationship between her eyes being open and her headaches? I didn't know what the problem was, I only knew what it wasn't. We hadn't come to the right

19

answer; we hadn't even come to the right question.

Medicine is frustrating like that. We want easy, quick, distinguished questions that result in smooth, easy, fixable answers. We have reduced the body to a study of the systems, independent from one another. The training of doctors has been divided into subspecialties in order to accommodate our need for ease of study and understanding. Unfortunately, this also feeds people's belief that there are fast, easy answers. The only real problem with all of this is that it isn't true. The body isn't a bunch of separate systems bound together under a boundary that we call the skin. Medicine isn't a separate set of systems that can be studied in isolation. Specialists who know only one part of the body or system often make medicine harder, not easier. In many instances, patients have several medical specialists working on separate parts of their bodies, who never talk to each other. It reminds me so much of the elephant being explored by the eight blind men. Each explores a given part of the elephant. Each describes their part eloquently but not one description matches another. A huge fight breaks out over which description is of the real elephant. Again, as in a play, the audience can see what is happening, yet can't fix the confusion.

Sarah was about to enter medical-specialist land. She had limited funds, so there was a great deal of reluctance on everyone's part to do lots of expensive diagnoses. She was so young that everyone rationalized that nothing terribly serious could be happening. Sarah began to fall apart, literally and figuratively speaking. She began to fall. A sprained ankle here, a fall and bruise there. She began having stomach problems, no doubt stress-related. Her headaches became so excessive she became suicidal. Her vision and her ability to describe it became so limited that she knew she was simply going crazy. There was an internist, a psychiatrist, a gastroenterologist, and an orthopedist on her case. All specialists described a piece, their piece, of this young woman. In total frustration, Sarah and I decided that she needed to see an ophthalmol-

20

ogist. Why not? Maybe one more specialist would give us a different vantage point of the elephant.

This move did not give us another vantage point, or another perspective. It gave us a diagnosis—macular degeneration. This young woman was going blind. Fast. She was right. Having her eyes open let in too much light, overstimulating the nerves and causing headaches. She fell because she couldn't see. She couldn't describe what she saw because it changed daily. She couldn't get a sense of it because it had never been a learned part of her. Her nausea was because she couldn't find and maintain a horizon. She couldn't find herself in space. Her proprioceptive capacity, how she found herself in relationship to the space and things around her, was failing her. Her other senses hadn't been able to adapt and keep up the pace of her loss of vision. She wasn't going crazy. She was going blind.

Sarah shifted with the diagnosis. She solidified. She went rafting on the Colorado River so she could see the Grand Canyon. She took out a loan so she could go to Europe and see famous buildings, paintings, and sculptures. She researched institutions of higher education that had the capacity to work with disabilities and headed back for a degree at a college in the Midwest that supported disabilities. She joined the National Federation of the Blind. She became an advocate and activist on behalf of other disabled students. She provided the voice that began forcing colleges and universities to adapt programs and policies to serve the disabled students who wanted to attend their schools, disabled students who wanted access to and on college campuses. She empowered herself. She wore sunglasses and visors to relieve her headaches. She learned braille, how to use a cane, and how to use a computer by touch. She climbed ladders to work with Habitat for Humanity in order to have a house of her own.

Fifteen years have now gone by. She is now about to begin the journey of using a guide dog. With hyper-mobile joints, learning to handle a guide dog is going to be a task. She talks about needing to bond to an animal in a way she has never even bonded to a person. She also is able to describe how daily she has periods of feeling like a young child, unable to care for herself. How those feelings require her to consider over and over again what it means to lose the boundaries of self. How each day is an opportunity to reinvent herself. A blessing and a curse.

Do I question that Sarah will continue to accomplish her life? No, not for one minute. Will she find herself a job that matches her tenacity? That's a much harder question. That question depends as much on society as on Sarah.

Don't Just Do Something, Stand There!
David

David was a CEO of a major corporation. He had seen me several times over a period of several years for this and that injury. He was driven. If he was in pain, he would manage to make and keep his appointments. I always got much of "the story" on the basis of whether he showed up or not. He was a large middle-aged man, slightly overweight, who tended to over-do it physically on the vacations he took. He would come in with complaints of back pain after playing thirty-six holes of golf for six days straight, after not having played for three years. He would come in with shoulder pain after taking a raft trip with his children for a week, having never rafted nor paddled a day, prior to the trip, in his life. As soon as his pain disappeared, he did too. There was never any follow-up, no exercises or strength program, no dedication to getting into shape before he took the next vacation. There were always words to that effect, but never any action. Reality always crept in, like light under a door jam, pushing the "what I want to do" into a far corner. He had too little time, too much money, and too many opportunities.

After one round of lumbar back pain, he made an appointment with his orthopedic physician. The doctor told him that he really needed to make some lifestyle changes. I asked him what the doctor said. He replied that the doctor had referred him to me, so that I would give him the hard bad news, and he needed to follow my instructions this time. I laughed. I told him he needed to exercise daily, lose fifty pounds, and limit his work schedule to sixty hours a week. Then, we both laughed! He was a wonderful guy.

This particular spring morning was different. David appeared with no appointment. Patients sometimes do that. They need reassurance, or connection, or an appointment. Somehow, physically coming into the office reinforces for them that it isn't such a bad place. Many times, their efforts toward compliance go up if they make the appointment in person rather than over the phone. In any case, and for whatever reason, David appeared. He sat down and waited nearly twenty minutes for me to appear out of one door on my way into another. This was enough out of character that it stopped me in my tracks.

To my knowledge, David had never voluntarily sat down for twenty minutes in the middle of the day, away from the business of making money. I pulled up a chair opposite him and asked what was going on.

His chief complaint was shoulder pain. The pain was intense and relentless. The pain was enough to change his sleep patterns. It was changing how he moved and held his arm. It was interfering with everyday life functions, like eating and opening doors. Any time pain causes that much change in a person's behavior, it is notable. He had seen his doctor, who had offered him a diagnosis of bursitis and had given him a cortisone injection.

I like cortisone. The fact that we produce it ourselves to alter the course of inflammation has always impressed me. One good cortisone shot in the hands of a skillful physician and a well-placed needle is, often as not, a miracle cure. With one well-placed cortisone shot, some good range of motion exercises and a follow-up strengthening program, many patients end up better in their entire body because of the bursitis.

I knew that there had been a shot, and a skillful doctor directing the needle. Knowing David, I was certain there still had been no follow-up, no range-of-motion activities, no strengthening program, and no re-evaluation. There was certainly work to be done. However, none of that was different, and none of it accounted for David coming, in person, sitting, and waiting in my office. Something else was wrong.

David looked genuinely worried. After answering questions along the lines of what makes it worse, what makes it better, what about the pain is causing you to be afraid, David said this was a pain he had never had before. It was deeper, or perhaps over a broader area, or perhaps it was so unusual, he really couldn't explain it to me at all. This caused him to worry. He was under a great deal of stress at work. This had led his internal medicine doctor to reassure him that it was a somatic problem and was not unusual under the circumstances.

Somatism. *Soma*, a Greek word meaning the body, as separate from the psyche. *Cis*, a Latin add-on to denote "on the near side of," closest to real, to make real. I've never been able to make any logical sense of this concept.

This concept wants us to believe that we can imagine something into our body that isn't really there. Since I've always believed we only have one body, and that our brain is a part of it, I haven't been able to figure out how our brain is outside of us enough to put something into the rest of us. Before a true "somatisizing" diagnosis works, a practitioner must buy into a mind/body split.

The mind/body concept is a philosophical one defined by Descartes. It is system separation. These are theoretical ideas that, while sounding plausible, functionally, aren't possible. When is the body not influenced by the brain? When is the brain not influenced by the body? When are the biochemicals in our body not influencing our brain and body as a unit?

I can understand fantasy. To pretend or mentally construct a non-reality into something that appears real. Animation (still pictures that appear to move) is certainly an example. Our eyes are happy to accept that the movement is occurring; when, in fact, these are drawings that are flipped rapidly enough that the illusion of movement occurs. The word nonsense makes perfect sense to me. *Non-sense.* It's tough to make sense out of nonsense. Fantasy is non-real.

Something felt or perceived is something felt or perceived. Those of us who sit outside the feeling or perception are not in a great position for observation. We cannot crawl behind someone else's skin and feel or perceive as they feel or perceive. Therefore, how on Earth can we be in a position to judge if their feelings or perceptions are real or not? Perhaps, some day a form of technology will exist that can do this, but we're not there yet.

David was in pain and worried about it. That was all the reality I needed to know. He was early for his appointment the next day, an "add-on" appointment that I had created for him at six-thirty in the morning. He was waiting in the hall when I arrived. The moment I felt his arm and hand, I knew something was wrong. His fingers didn't respond evenly to movement. His skin was pale and lacked vitality. His muscles were tense and unresponsive. There was noticeable atrophy in the deltoid muscles (the muscles that wrap and make up the contour of the shoulder). He couldn't point to the pain. It was elusive, too elusive for him to find the pain inside himself. I now understood differently why he was worried.

Pain is tough. For one thing, we have a word for something that has many forms. When someone tells me they are in pain it is next to meaningless. Is it hot, sharp, dull, knifelike, "toothache" like? Is the pain localized or diffuse, restless, or migrating? Are the descriptors the patient chooses the same as the images I have when they use a certain word?

Pain is a perception. We now know that different people have different thresholds of pain and different numbers of pain receptors. There are many different chemicals a body can utilize as pain mitigators. These chemicals change the form, function, or awareness of the pain. We all respond to pain medications differently, because of these basic physiological differences. I suspect many of the differences are genetic, and we cannot simply "choose" to experience pain one way or another. That means as long as we are separate humans, we cannot fully understand what is meant by the word "pain." No matter how well I listen or how hard I try, I cannot know if my interpretation of the words someone uses and their experience is similar to the words I would chose and my own experience of pain. The best we can hope for is an acknowledgment that something is awry.

Pain also has different meanings for different people. Some people are socially and culturally allowed to have pain, therefore they report all of it. Others are not. By the time they report any pain at all, they are in serious pain. I am afraid we are all afraid of pain. As practitioners, we tend to underestimate it. As patients, more often than not, we underreport it. I haven't spoken directly with God about this yet, but I don't think there are rewards in heaven for tolerating pain. I believe it is a warning service plain and simple. Sometimes, we can listen to our warnings at the beginning, the very nuance, of the pain data. Other times, our bodies have to hit us over the head with an iron frying pan before we notice anything at all.

David needed additional diagnoses. The question was which specialist should he see? I chose neurology. David was examined. I received a lengthy report back with a treatment plan. We launched on task. This time, David followed through. He made time to swim. He stretched. He did the very specific exercises to counteract the atrophy in his shoulder and arm. I measured, I massaged, I passively worked his range of motion. We worked together. Nothing worked. Four weeks went by. We were losing ground. The muscle atrophy was more pronounced, not less. His ability to accurately move his arm and hand had decreased, not increased. He went back to the neurologist. This time, I wanted an MRI.

MRIs, CT scans, PET scans, and SPECT scans are the

biggest "good news, bad news" technology I know. The fact that we can put a person into a giant electromagnet and watch every cell move and create a computer-enhanced view of that action is nothing short of incredible. The fact that we can "see" at a cellular level is a marvel, but sometimes, the data are not what we hope for.

For the most part, I believe data are just data. There are no "bad data." Information is, after all, only information. We don't have to act on all information. It doesn't demand anything of us, per se. Data are just data. I like data. I am an information junkie. Sometimes, though, the data we get is more than we want to know. In this case, the MRI showed a rather large astroglioma; a very fast growing, highly spreadable cancer of the brain.

David took the information in stride. He did far better than I did. He said he was eternally grateful to know that something really was wrong, and why it was so different for him. It also propelled him to San Francisco, where he, supported by his wife, underwent the latest in experimental brain surgery, chemotherapy, and radiation. His wife was as isolated as he was. They had left their children home with a nanny. She called several times weekly, in fear and frustration. They found themselves in a teaching, experimental medical model. Although wonderful for what society learns from all that happens in these institutions, for patients and their families sitting in the rooms and waiting areas, isolated from their support systems, they are still institutions.

Teaching hospitals are not great places to get lots of well-articulated information and support. Teaching hospitals are where students learn the language and lingo that separate doctors from patients. It is, in practice, not in the teaching hospital, that good doctors learn to set aside medical linguistics for honest direct answers and an adequate dose of hand-holding.

Being separated from family and friends in a medical crisis is extremely difficult. It is in those times that we need context and consistency. We need to be supported by those who can read us clearly and with ease. It is at times of crisis when we need people who already hold us as intimates. We need access to those who can hold us as we cry. We need the bracing and embracing that having family, friends, and community is all about. In times of medical crisis we need those we trust the most to provide questions and perspectives. We need humor and memories in a delicate balance with tears and grief.

If the teaching, experimenting hospital is in our own community and does not require that we leave family and friends, the coolness of the institution can be overcome. Away from support systems, the institution becomes inhumane all too often.

Three months and thousands of dollars later, they came home . . . to wait. David was too ill to be coming into the clinic, so I went to his home. We needed to adapt their home for care. Home is where he wanted to be. For a man who was seldom home in his "well" life, he was dedicated to being at home in his "ill" life. This created a multi-faceted problem. There were the roll-up-the-throw-rugs-and-bring-in-the-commode problems. There were the how-do-we-move-a-big-man-with-little, and some days, no capacity to move himself. More importantly, an entire family had to make a person who had been absent for much of their lives the absolute center of their existence. The level of adaptation that this required of everyone was amazing. Every family member had learning to do, from learning safe transfer techniques, to the anticipation of what changes in their environment were needed to make it safe for David's new needs, to the purchase of baby food to offer him multiple food choices. Adaptations were required not only of David, but of every family member.

One afternoon, David and I were working together. I was moving limbs that were unresponsive. His circulation was poor. Swelling was now present in every joint. His pain levels were climbing beyond his ability to manage, yet he refused the pain medications because they made him "lose his mind." He was working hard on the final stages of getting his family and business affairs in order. There were meetings with business partners, lawyers, financial advisors. He needed his brain.

Each of these meetings took huge amounts of energy. They not only involved hard intellectual work, but they were emotionally grueling. The meeting which had occurred just prior to my coming for our therapy session was with his business partners. David began our conversation reflecting on how it felt to him that they were all so angry at him. He simply couldn't understand what he had done to them. He could not understand why his business partners would respond with anger. He wanted them to treat him with respect and dignity. I laughed and pointed out that he was slightly out of the typical board room attire, as he was holding these meetings propped up in bed in his loose fitting pajamas. The partners sat on the bed or in straight-backed chairs that were brought in from the dining room. He reflected for a few minutes and then said, "You know, Sue, this is a terrible mess I've gotten everyone into." I was stunned. I wondered aloud how he thought he had "created" the tumor in his brain. David said, "Well, I must have. It's my brain. Everyone is acting like I got sick just to ruin their lives or get back at them."

Anger is part of any change process when the change is thrust upon us, especially if the change is against our will, or out of our control. I can't begin to count the number of times anger has been my response. Myself as a parent being angry at something as small as a child who would not brush his teeth in a timely enough manner that he could be whisked out the door to child care or school quickly enough to support my work schedule. The child and I would both end up angry. We were both out of control . . . out of control of the clock, the time requirements, the requirements themselves. Other times, the same activity of teeth-brushing provoked no anger as there were no time constraints. Confusing as it seems, it is a natural response.

Anger is a biochemical reaction to threat. It was built into us long ago and far away as a survival mechanism. It propels us to fight, to flee, or to freeze. It readies us to meet danger head on, with all of our senses on alert. It increases our oxygen levels, heart rate, and blood flow. It alerts our brains, and opens the storage areas in our body, which hold extra nutrient sources. Anger, and its bio-chemical messengers, are our disaster-preparedness team. Just being or feeling out of control propels us headlong into this rush of survival rage. Our jungles are different. Our threats are no longer actual predators. They are, however, still jungles. We still feel very vulnerable and in danger.

In David's world, everyone was being asked to gear up. To get ready to do without him, his intellect, contacts, money, expertise, personality, and solid leadership. All were having to face their new responsibilities. Would they be as competent as he in the facet of work or family that they were forced to take over? They had no control over what was happening to them, and they hadn't asked for any of these changes. It is a human condition to be angry. Angry, blaming, and shaming. Far better to make him the target of our uncertainties than ourselves.

We like blame in our society. Somebody or something is always to blame. Something caused these changes. If it wasn't them, then it must be David. We blame patients all too often. Perhaps they weren't working hard enough to take care of themselves, or taking their medications properly. The patients might be lying to us or to themselves about whether or not the signs or symptoms are real. We build a case that they had somehow "earned the dis-ease" or "created the injury." We accuse the patient of magical thinking and then go right on and do it ourselves as practitioners. We just don't like to fail. Some find themselves blaming God in sit-uations like these, others blame themselves. Still others blame

31

"bugs," or pathogens. We want control and we want explanations! Humans have always behaved like this. We can look to anthropology and find that, throughout the ages, humankind has invented stories, gods, enemies, and myths for explaining the unexplainable.

Personally, I like to blame the planet. If we live on the earth, there are four rules, based on Newton's laws of gravity:

1. Something at rest tends to stay there, unless something else hits it.
2. The direction and intensity it moves is directly related to what hits it.
3. For every action, there is an equal and opposite reaction.
4. Gravity is relentless.

Those are the rules. They are basic laws of physics. They apply to everything, animate and inanimate alike. They apply to relationships. They apply at all times and in all places, regardless of how important, or how different. We can change the rules, but we have to change planets to do so. Many of us spend more time pretending that we live on another planet than we do accepting the rules. There is a great deal of freedom in these rules. If we accept them, we can predict quite even-handedly how things are apt to go. On this planet, if we fall, we don't have to ponder which direction we're going to fall.

David and everyone around him were deep into the rules. Everything was going along just fine, until a brain tumor hit David. How fast and in what direction David and his family moved was directly related to the severity of the tumor. David's need to move away from his business and family meant others had to move closer in order to fill his space. David was dying. David was falling down.

David's medical care was now being done long distance and

over the phone. A local neuro-oncologist was named to do medication support, but he was unfamiliar with the treatments David had received. The doctors in San Francisco weren't here to see David's changes. David was sinking, fast. By telephone, the doctors were telling the family that everything was just fine. Surely, the family was just imagining the worst. Often chemotherapy is hard on patients, so perhaps that was what was making him so ill. The local doctors didn't want to disagree with the providers of the treatment. The family was not supported in trusting their own instincts. They were not being sustained or empowered to see and feel what they actually saw and felt. There was no shared reality.

Three days before Christmas, David's oldest son announced that he was going skiing and would be gone several days. He had had enough. As the oldest teenager, and a strong healthy athlete, much of the moving of David had fallen on his broad shoulders. Distance is a vital way to find new perspective.

In times of trouble or stress, I have often headed for a hike to the highest surrounding hills in order to find a new view. Often the panoramic view literally opens my head to new insights. I was sure that this teenager needed not only some recreation time, but also a new perspective. The greater issue was the timing of his trip.

His mom was terrified that she and the two younger children could not handle David. She was fearful that they would fall attempting to move David. *She was afraid.* She was worried about a teenager heading off to the hills without specific plans of where, for how long, or with whom. She was worried about a teenager driving in holiday traffic on ice-covered roads. She was already dealing with enough loss. A family meeting was called. All of these issues and more were aired. I told the eldest son that I was sure his father was in the final stages of dying. He quietly, but persistently, explained to me that if the oncology specialists said that he wasn't dying, he wasn't dying.

A compromise was reached. He was to sit with his father for an hour while his mom went out to do a little Christmas shopping. He was also to find a friend to go skiing with who could share the driving. They were expected to return by dinner that same night. I agreed to stay to help with transfers and care. I also got on the phone to every nurse friend I knew to see if we could find some night relief for a couple of nights. It was clear this entire family was on the edge. It was Christmas week, the probabilities of finding hired help were slight. Since no doctor would agree that David was sinking this quickly, hospice care had not been ordered. Denial defined the medical establishment. Denial left this family in crisis to fend for itself.

I often wonder if medical professionals ever fully understand the authority patients and families turn over to them. I wonder if a physician is aware of the depth of the consequences when we tell a patient's family, "Your father is not dying." Words are spoken as if they are truth. Spoken as if there is control. Spoken as if humans can actually predict the future.

As a child, I realized that I could not throw a series of stones into a lake or pond far enough that the ripples of one stone would not overlap the ripples of the others. It was beyond my physical limit to throw a stone so far, there would not be interaction. It was a powerful lesson delivered to me by physics at age seven. Can we, as health-care practitioners, learn that each word is like a stone thrown into a still pond? The ripples will happen. They will over-lap.

Failure of a treatment to work is not something we take lightly as practitioners. We like things to work. The vast majority of people in medicine are dedicated hard-working professionals who are in the field to help people. Sometimes, it doesn't appear that way because we get caught up in the treatment instead of remaining focused on the patient.

On Christmas Eve day, David's wife called me at home in a

panic. David was having difficulty breathing. She couldn't get anyone on the phone in San Francisco. The oncologist on call in town knew nothing about the case personally so deferred to the doctors in San Francisco. I told her to dial 911 and transport him to the closest hospital. The hospital on-call oncologist, who knew absolutely nothing about the case, admitted him. He stood by all night. He explained to the entire family that David was close to death, and that there was nothing more that could be done other than measures for comfort. I have often said that the opposite of "Just don't stand there, *Do* something," is, "Don't just *Do* something, *stand there!*" This physician was able to stand there. The entire family stood by. The children were all able to say good-by before David lapsed into a profound coma. David died on Christmas Day.

Christmas is no longer the same for anyone in that family. Years have gone by. The lack of nurture in this story affected David and his entire family profoundly. The failure of a treatment and the failure to acknowledge reality combined to create a greater failure for a whole family. The failure to acknowledge reality on the part of the medical professionals created a loss of faith as great as the loss of David. It created a failure for the entire family to believe in medicine, in treatment, in medical professional judgment. These wounds in human spirit and emotion will take more then years and medicine to heal. It is around this profound lack of shared reality that alternative medicine nowadays is evident. It is this lack of shared reality that created the myths of the past. If you can't make sense of it, make up a story.

Apollo, as it turns out, didn't really drive the sun across the sky each morning. Myths die much harder than people. A popular medical myth is that practitioners are gods . . . medical gods who can drive the demons of disease away. Death is hard. Sometimes, to remain living, is even harder . . . especially when medical professionals fail to adapt and to notice the living. The family members needed as much healing and treatment as the patient. We didn't establish a medical myth for now to heal those who would remain living in David's life.

Dying on Planet Earth
Harold

Harold had just turned eighty-two and was suffering from back pain when he was referred to my office by his internal medicine specialist. His intake card was pretty sparsely filled out. He listed a few medications, a previously broken shoulder that had been surgically repaired, an old World War II injury to a knee, and a "bad sacroiliac pain." As I glanced over his intake information I thought to myself, "*Not bad. Hope I am doing this well at his age.*"

Harold was about as illuminating in person as he was on his intake card. When I asked him how he was, he replied, "I'm in pretty good shape, for the shape I'm in!" When I asked why his doctor had referred him to me, he replied, "The pain in my back." When I asked Harold how much his back hurt, he replied, "Not that much." I could see that our communication had to have "enhancement" before we were going to end up being a "team."

Harold turned out to be quite a story-teller. He would go on and on about nearly any subject, including sports, where in the world he had traveled, his opinions on politics, or his exercise program. There was little information about his problem or pain. His back told tales of its own, however.

Harold's muscles were tight and short. His face winced as I touched areas of tension and spasm, but his words never revealed anything. The range of motion within his spinal column, at his pelvis, and at his hip joints was very limited. Most eighty-plus-year-olds have stiff muscles and limited range of motion. Harold was in excellent shape, however, so his limited range of motion was a bit surprising.

I attempted to search for more information throughout the session. When had his pain started? Was there a change in exercise program or activity that had preceded his pain? Had he ever had pain like this before? Were there activities that made it better or worse? What had he done to take care of the pain in his back himself? Was there any other sign or symptom that he could think of that might be related? Each question produced little data, and another story. I was beginning to think that what Harold needed most was an active listener, and perhaps back pain was going to find him one.

The more I poked and prodded, the more Harold winced and told stories. I wanted him to talk less and tell me more, he wanted me to poke less and listen more. We were getting nowhere fast.

An hour later I wrote out a regime of stretching, ice, and anti-inflammatory medications. As I was reviewing my instructions, I got my first real piece of information. Harold told me he couldn't take any more of "those pills," as they made him sick to his stomach. I pursued this one piece of incomplete information like a hungry dog.

"Does it make your stomach ache, or do you feel nauseated?" I asked.

"No," he replied. "I throw up."

"How long have you taken these pills in the past?" I asked.

"Once or twice," he responded.

"Once or twice?" I said. "I meant how many days did you take them before they made you ill?"

"Like I said, I only took them once or twice, and then I threw up," he replied.

"Are you saying that you threw up with only one pill?" I asked for further clarification.

38

"That's right," he said, "I hate those damn things, because I hate to throw up."

I wanted to start the entire hour all over again from the beginning. I had patients lined up on my schedule all day, a list of phone calls, and reports to write, so I simply did not have the time to follow up. I drew a line through the anti-inflammatory medication and wrote a note to myself to follow up with his internal medicine physician. I wanted to know what his doctor knew about Harold's stomach, intestines, and blood work.

The next day, I spoke with Harold's physician. I did not learn a great deal more. Harold had received two prescriptions for anti-inflammatory medications in the past. He had filled the prescriptions and had never complained to his doctor about any problem. There were no chart notes about gut pain or related problems. There had been routine blood work done, showing nothing of significance.

Harold came back in two weeks later. He had followed the stretching and ice instructions perfectly. He was more limber, had less spasms, and no change in pain whatsoever. In fact, Harold reported that, if anything, his pain was worse. Perplexing. Several stories later, Harold dropped one more diamond of information.

"I think that ice on my back makes me pee more," said Harold.

"Really," I responded. "That's very interesting. What makes you think so?"

"Well, every time I ice my back, I pee. Then I pee a lot for several hours after I ice my back," he said.

"Could it be that you are drinking more water?" I asked. I push increasing water intake to my patients to the point that it becomes a joke.

"No, I've been drinking lots of water for some time now, I'm always thirsty," he replied firmly. "It's the ice."

With the three pieces of information I had about Harold, back pain, stomach pain with even small doses of non-steroidal anti-inflammatory medication, and increased thirst and urine output, I was ready to refer Harold back to his primary health-care provider for a fasting glucose tolerance test. I was beginning to think that Harold's back pain was not about Harold's back, but rather about his pancreas. The ordered test showed Harold's urine was positive for sugar.

Diabetes Mellitus was first described by a Roman physician in A.D. 2 as a "melting down of the flesh and bones into urine." Diabetes means "running through." Mellitus means "honey." Diabetes Mellitus, or diabetes, as we usually refer to it, describes a condition where there is an unusual outpouring of urine containing sugar. This comes from a time in medicine when urine was both smelled and tasted as part of any diagnosis. The urine of a diabetic patient would still smell and taste sweet today. Thankfully, however, today we learn the sugar content by chemical analysis.

There was a time in medical history when diabetes was misunderstood as a kidney disease because of the outpouring of urine. Physicians thought the kidneys were malfunctioning. As our understanding of the physiology of the body increased, we realized that it was a disorder in the way carbohydrates were utilized by the tissues of the body. Before carbohydrates can be used by the body as energy, they must be broken down by an enzyme, insulin, that is produced and stored in the pancreas. There is still a great deal to learn about diabetes today. Every year, both our understanding and our ability to treat this disease changes. If a body cannot utilize the carbohydrates in food, it will use first our fat stores and then our protein, such as muscle, as food. The result is increased urine, excessive thirst, hunger, and weight loss, and ultimately, death. This entire process in A.D. 2 did not take long.

My perspective of Harold as being "in good shape" by not being overweight, being of lean muscle mass, and already well trained in drinking plenty of water, were all, in fact, signs not of his good health, but of a poorly functioning pancreas.

Harold's physician began treatment for diabetes. Harold's back got better with insulin. His back pain reduced substantially as his blood sugar got under control. We agreed to stay in touch on his exercise and stretching program. Harold took great pride in his muscles at eighty-two. I figured the least I could do was help him "stay in good shape for the shape he was in."

A couple of months went by before I heard from Harold that his back pain had returned. He came back in so I could review his exercise and stretching program. I thought he had no doubt "overdone" some facet. When Harold appeared, I was shocked. He had lost a good deal more weight. I questioned him about his eating, his blood sugar, and his exercise. His physician had told him that as long as his blood sugar stayed within safe ranges, he would not need to see him for six months. Harold's doctor had not listed weight loss as a problem, so Harold hadn't given it much thought. He certainly had not given it any worry-time.

We modified his exercise program, and I sent him back to his primary physician for immediate follow-up. This diagnosis had seemed so straightforward that I could not understand what the problem was. He had shown me his carefully kept blood-sugar record, and nothing had leapt out from the pages at me. Perhaps a change in the form or quantity of insulin medications needed to be made or a change in his diet.

Harold did not make it to his follow-up appointment. His wife called me late in the afternoon on the Friday of the same week I had seen him. He had fallen down ten stairs at home and they were at the emergency room. Harold was complaining of very sharp back pain and difficulty breathing. His primary physician could not be reached, and the emergency room physician had carefully explained that anything they did had to be pre-approved by either the insurance company or Harold's primary physician. The insurance company offices were now closed, so until Harold's physician or the on-call physician could be reached, nothing could be done as Harold was technically "medically stable." Harold's wife was frantic. She had never heard him complain of such pain. I was certain she was telling the truth.

By the time I arrived at the hospital, Harold's primary care medical office had identified the on-call physician. The on-call physician had never met Harold, but had ordered a set of X-rays and some blood work.

The X-ray showed that Harold had broken three ribs at their attachment to the vertebrae. This would certainly account for Harold's "stabbing" back pain. The blood work showed very high blood-sugar levels. Harold admitted to me that he had felt light-headed when he began falling down the stairs.

I questioned him at length about his insulin medication schedule. Harold insisted that he had not missed or been late in a dose. Looking over his carefully kept book, I believed him. The piece of information that stuck out immediately as I looked at his book was the change in writing. Early in the week, it had been solid and perfectly written. The day before it looked shaky. The three entries on this day were barely legible.

I reviewed the X-ray. The breaks themselves were clean. The bones were frothy and very grey. The Roman physician's description of diabetes in A.D. 2 entered my mind, *The melting down of flesh and bone to urine.* Harold's bones were "melting" away. We refer to this today as bone density. Harold's bone looked more like meringue than bone. Once again, I was beginning to have second thoughts about the diagnosis.

Harold was admitted to the hospital. His insulin levels had to get under control and his pain had to be addressed. I left wondering what the next day was going to bring.

I visited him on my way to the office early the next morning.

Harold was sitting up. As I entered the room, I thought at first it was because he felt better. The moment I saw his face, I knew otherwise. His eyes were closed, his brow furrowed, and his mouth was taunt with a grimace. Harold was in pain.

I spoke to him, asking how his night had been. He said that he had not slept, sitting was the only position in which he could get even a little breath in, and that his coughing hurt so badly, that he wanted to die. Up to that moment, I had heard nothing about a "cough." I asked for a description of his cough. Harold reported that it had started about two that morning. It felt like his chest was on fire and he had stabbing pain in his back and belly each time he coughed. I asked if the pain medication had helped at all. He said he hadn't had any because every time they gave him a pain pill he threw it up. He refused the pills after vomiting twice because it hurt so much to vomit. He decided to just live with the pain. *Or die with it*, I thought to myself as I left the room to see if Harold's reported information matched the chart notes. It did.

I left a note asking the physician on-call for Harold's doctor to give me a call. I felt we needed to know what was really happening. I knew he was going to need a scan to give us the information we needed. I was not sure that we were any better off in the twentieth century in medicine, than we were in the first century.

I needed to help Harold be free of pain. I wasn't sure what was going on or what his correct diagnosis was going to be. I did know that if Harold couldn't take deeper breaths, get some sleep, and eat, soon, it wouldn't make any difference *what* the diagnosis was. Harold was going to be dead of pneumonia . . . Harold was going to be dead of pain.

An MRI was ordered. Harold had a mass on his pancreas, liver, and stomach. An exploratory surgery was ordered. The surgeon was young enough to be my child. I smiled as I thought about how funny it was to be middle-aged—old enough to still feel young, old enough to recognize that your children could replace you.

43

The surgeon came in to introduce himself to Harold and his wife. He carefully outlined the process and procedure. As he got up to leave, Harold stopped him as he approached the door. He said, "Doctor, if you find I am full of cancer, I want you to just sew me up and do nothing at all." The surgeon asked Harold if he understood what that would mean. Harold said he did. The surgeon also asked if Harold had an advance directive that he and his wife had discussed. Harold said that he did. The surgeon asked to see it. Harold's wife pulled a copy out of her purse. The surgeon asked to have it placed in Harold's medical file, and assured Harold that his directions and directives would be followed. An hour later, Harold was in surgery.

The surgery lasted only thirty minutes. Harold's wife was excited as the surgeon rounded the corner. She felt it must have gone very well. I had a sinking feeling in my stomach. I knew it hadn't. Harold had also known.

Harold awoke in his hospital room. His wife was waiting for him to awake. When he asked what they had found, she began to cry and couldn't answer. I told Harold the surgeon would be up in a few minutes and that we would all talk about it then. Harold looked me in the eye and said, "It wasn't good, was it?" "No," I replied solemnly. "Well," he said, "then as soon as we get this pain under control, I want to go home and get busy saying my good-byes."

I told Harold that he had been put on a morphine drip pump. A device that the patient has control over. With it, patients can give as little or as much pain medicine as they feel necessary. The pump would not allow an overdose. I asked if Harold was in pain. He said that he was. I showed him how to use the pump. By the time the surgeon came in to talk, Harold was vomiting. Harold's system did not like much in the way of medication.

Pain management has changed drastically in the last decade. Our understanding of pain and the process of addiction is in great part responsible for the changes. The other part is played by the wide variety of new medications available. We have become more adept at combining medications and more aware of dosage requirements to keep pain under control. Lastly, a new set of surgical pain interventions is nothing short of miraculous. It takes a good pain management physician and team to consider all of the possible ways to address pain. This is a medical specialty in and of itself.

It was obvious to everyone involved in Harold's care that management of his pain was not going to be by medication. In the hospital, we could administer other anti-nausea/vomiting medications to counter act the post surgical pain medications needed. Managing his pain in that way over a longer period of time was less than perfect. The surgeon and I both felt a referral to a pain clinic and consideration of a surgical procedure, in Harold's case a celiac plexus nerve block, might be the best option.

Within a few days, Harold was ready for his second surgical procedure. This one was to kill the nerves to the cancer-affected organs. This would allow Harold to be pain-free. We all hoped this would allow him to go about his life, at the end of his life, as he would want. This surgery lasted forty-five minutes. Harold was ready for a small meal shortly afterward. He was on his way home within hours.

Harold and his wife had requested hospice support. Hospice is such a wonderful way to be fully supported professionally and personally at the end of life. It provides not only the daily care and nursing needs of the patient, but also the emotional and, in many cases, the respite needs for the family. Hospice professionals are carefully selected and trained to provide the "caring" that every dying human deserves. The hospice team trains family members to take "medical care" of their loved one, and to consider changes and adaptations that need to be made in the home so that the person dying can remain there. In many communities, not only does hospice analyze the needs, it provides the carpenters to make the adaptations. It truly is a support system designed to work. In most cases, it costs far less than caring for the dying individual in a hospital or nursing home setting. Most patients far prefer to remain at home, provided they don't feel like a major burden on their family. With hospice in place, there is no need to feel like a burden. Patients can feel like a gift.

Harold lived another six weeks. He invited extended friends and family members to visit, either in person or by phone. Because he was not cognitively affected by pain medication, he was able to be present for each and every one of those good-byes. He and his wife were able to make last-minute changes in their trust. He executed his own legal document changes. He walked, talked, told stories, held his grandchildren, ate his favorite foods (although usually in one bite quantities), enjoyed his favorite sports programs, and his garden. On one visit, just one week before he died, he walked out to his garden to pick his blueberries with me. He insisted that he wanted me to take them home to my family.

Harold died quietly, in his own bed, surrounded by a limited amount of medical intervention and equipment. The medical supplies he had surrounding him were for comfort only. They were not unsightly tubes or frightening blips and beepers that made death seem like something from another planet.

Harold died on planet Earth. He had the loving care of his family and professionals who were determined to make him comfortable. He was able to live his dying because of modern surgical medicine and a truly advanced pain management team.

Driving Miss Cathy Back to Life
Cathy

Rehabilitation medicine is an interesting mix of odds and ends. "*Re*" is a Latin word meaning to do again, indicating repetition, to go back and forth. *Habil* comes from an ancient Latin word, *habilis*, meaning able, skillful, to make ready for occupancy. Thus, we have such words as habit, habitate, habitat. *Habilitate* literally means to clothe, or equip. If we add the suffix '*tion*,' making it rehabilitation, it means we are in a process of "doing" the equipping. If we make the ending the suffix '*ed*,' the word becomes rehabilitated, and we are done! That is perhaps why practitioners drawn to "rehab" medicine, in whatever form or training model, presume that their practice of medicine will be a *process* rather than a *fixing*. "Rehab" medicine is not a quick fix practice. The process of healing we enter into with patients is for the long haul. We may get done, but by definition, we may just get to do "it" over and over and over again. We don't have a "fix" definition. We have a maintenance definition. This really makes a lot of difference in how we approach patients in general.

I suggest this in the relation to the story of Cathy, because Cathy is a perfect "good news, bad news" story. She came to me as an iatrogenic patient. *Iatros* is a Greek word, meaning healer, from '*io*' a Greek verb meaning to heal. *Iatrogenic* literally means a disease with a "genesis," or beginning, from the healer. Cathy was sick. She went to a physician. By the time he was finished treating her, she was severely ill.

Cathy was a college professor when she caught some form of a virus. She had a panic disorder all of her life. Prior to the virus, she was able to cope with her panic disorder and lived an unmedicated and functional life. For some reason, her body went ballistic in response to this particular pathogen. This happens. Perhaps over the next several decades, we'll have a better understanding of why. Right now, we don't know why. Instead of getting a little bit sick for a short period of time, Cathy got very sick over an extended period of time. Between having an extended illness and a panic disorder that escalated her illness, she became very dysfunctional. She worried that she was about to die. She worried that no one would be able to figure out what was wrong with her. She worried that she would get other illnesses if she was around other people. She worried that she would give her illness to students. All in all, her panic responses sent her to bed, where she stayed untreated for five years.

Five years is a long time to be in bed. She ate macaroni and cheese and drank juice and water. Someone came in to cook and clean. Otherwise, she saw no one, did nothing, and hid, usually in bed. Her friends disappeared, slowly, but steadily. With the help of her computer and the availability of the Internet, she began to do research on what might be wrong. "Good news, bad news. . . . " At some point in time, she talked herself into having three primary diseases, all self-diagnosed. She had Fibromyalgia. She had Chronic Fatigue. She had Chronic Fatigue Immune Deficiency Syndrome, commonly known as CFIDS. She had pain, she had lethargy, she had changes in her consciousness. Her symptoms fit CFIDS best. She settled on that.

The differences between signs and symptoms are significant. If there is a sign, other people know and can verify that it is there. An elevated fever is a good example of a sign. Thermometer in, thermometer out, and a reading is taken. As long as no one shakes down the thermometer or in the case of the new digital ones, resets it, any number of people can read the same numbers. Theoretically, with similar training, all medical practitioners who are trained to hear, see, feel, or smell something that is significant can all come up with the same information. Theoretically, if five physicians are in the same room at the same time and listen to the lungs of the same patient, they will all hear the same sounds. We know from experience that this isn't the case. Some people are just better at some skills than others, regardless of a similar knowledge base. At the very least, it is likely that several physicians would interpret the same sounds, sights, smells, and touch differently.

A symptom is something the patient feels inside themselves and describes to us. We do not expect a physician to feel what the patient feels. We record these as symptoms in our charts beginning with the words, "Patient reports," denoting that the patient has given us these pieces of information. Signs, on the other hand, we report as "findings."

Fibromyalgia, Chronic Fatigue, and CFIDS are syndromes. A syndrome is a condition defined by combining a set of signs and symptoms. These are hard diseases to quantify. There isn't a lab test or a temperature change, or a simple picture, we can take that shows that it is there. These diseases are elusive. Patients without panic disorders get "panicky" when their bodies are performing poorly, are hurt, and can't be easily "fixed." With a panic disorder, these diseases are compounded in extraordinary ways.

At the urging of a friend, Cathy was taken to a doctor who specialized in CFIDS. The complexity of this disease is staggering. Why a physician would want to specialize in it, outside of a research setting, is in and of itself questionable.

In order to get herself out of the house, Cathy had to blindfold herself, lie in the back seat of the friend's car, and cover herself snugly with a blanket. With a mask on her nose and mouth, led by a friend on either side, she made her way into the physician's office. The physician saw her for half an hour. He knew exactly what she needed—lots of supplements, which he could provide right there at his office, at prices that were much higher than the corner grocery store, and a combination of hydrocortisone and prednisone. Not a little medication, but a lot of medication, which he happily supplied by phone, year after year, without ever seeing this patient again.

I like cortisone. We produce it in our own bodies. It works. At these amounts, Cathy had been prescribed and over long periods of time, cortisone becomes dangerous and even lethal. Cathy developed the standard "cushionoid syndrome." She became very endemic (swollen) throughout her body. She couldn't move. She could swallow her several handfuls of pills each day but had little appetite for anything more. She was severely dysfunctional at this point. Five more years had gone by.

I had seen Cathy twelve years earlier for a sprained ankle. At that time, she was small, slight, bright-eyed, fast-talking, and had a clever wit. She was so rapid fire with words that unless I was very careful with the words I chose, she would make a pun out of everything. Her area of expertise was the classics. She was well-read and a delightful conversationalist.

While rehabilitating an ankle, correcting gait, and planning strengthening exercise programs, there are lots of opportunities for just plain conversation. The repetitious parts of a course of treatment often involve long periods of silence. This can be pretty boring. As a result of having time for conversation, my patients have educated me on numerous subjects. My definition of trivia is knowing more and more about less and less. I am sure every patient has contributed to my children all being trivia buffs. They have had to tolerate my never-ending reports of daily accumulated trivial data being shared at the dinner table! Cathy was good for this sort of thing and I had enjoyed working with her very much.

When the phone message came in to call her, I frankly couldn't place this person. Twelve years is about fifteen thousand patient visits later. I dug the old records out of the basement storage file cabinet and had done my best to glean a picture of this human, but it was not forthcoming. Speaking with her on the telephone was no help in my attempts to place her. On the telephone, she was sluggish sounding. She sounded underwater. She was, in fact, under water. The water that her own body was producing and withholding due to the drugs. We call these signs Cushinoid.

In our conversation, it became obvious that she could not come into the office. I could not determine what should or could be done without seeing her. I asked her to write down everything that she was putting into her mouth and I set up a time to see her in a few days.

I knocked on her front door. The yard and house were very tidy. From her helm in her bed, she ran one tight ship. It was obvious the students that she hired to care for her and her home were very respectful and kind. They were all doing a great job. Her pride had not been broken, only her health. I could barely discern the outline of her body in her darkened room (sunlight made her hurt). She blended into the bed pillows. She looked like a cross between the marshmallow man and the Pillsbury Dough Boy. We can laugh about it now. At the time, I was so upset, I nearly cried. I had to work very hard at imagining who this person was over a decade before. I had to sift through the haunts of my mental images to make anything fit. She looked familiar, but only in that obtuse sort of way. I likened it to the experience of seeing a perfect stranger on a street corner or in a crowd, and turning to glance again, thinking that they look like someone I've known.

Our interview could last only a few minutes. Conversation for Cathy was exhausting. I looked over her body. Pitting edema was everywhere. I guessed at the time she had twenty pounds of water weight. We had no way to tell, because although she owned a scale, her balance was so bad she couldn't step on it. We had to get her off the cortisone. We had to get her medicated for the panic disorder. We had to get her moving. We had to get her to eat. We had to get her weaned off the millions of pills on her kitchen shelf. We had so many things to do, I couldn't even begin to sort out how to begin!

I was too angry to speak with the physician who had created this mess. I called a psychiatric colleague at the medical school in town, and with him and an internist at the medical school satellite clinic close to her house, the three of us began to draw up a treatment plan, or in this case, a de-treatment plan. We had no idea what might be right or wrong with Cathy's health because she was sealed in a shell of excessive anti-inflammatory medications. We would have to play that by ear. What we did know was that we had to empower her to take control of her life, giving her the ability to slowly come off the cortisone and go on the anti-panic, anti-depression medications. This task is so tricky that in many cases, people fail. They just can't maintain their life through the physiological changes that are required. They either end up back on the drugs, or die. She had to buy into the program. We could and would stand by, but she had to do this one.

It has taken nearly two years to very slowly drop the hydro-cortisone and prednisone. The vitamins and supplements are nearly all gone. She eats real food. She has, in the last few months, begun to prepare food and cook for herself. She dusted off old recipes that she enjoyed over a decade ago. She had a birthday party this year, the first one in twelve years. She heard her god-daughter play a violin, the first music she has been able to hear without the barrier of ear plugs in over a decade.

She sleeps, she eats, she walks, she talks, she laughs, she cries, and she is now really angry! All the daily occurrences we all take for granted she lost for ten years. Her exercise is still limited to walking around her house and garden, up one set of stairs, and doing exercises holding cans of tuna fish as weights, but it is a start. She has lost fifteen pounds and has purchased the first articles of clothing in more than a decade.

Utilizing a psychology graduate student, we are beginning to desensitize her to the outside world she hasn't seen in over a decade. Cathy sweetly calls her time edging her way back into civilization, "Driving Miss Cathy." Together, twice a week, the graduate student introduces her to another aspect of society. Everyday experiences like how to use a credit card. Driving on roads that didn't exist when she quit driving a decade ago, she has to seek out landmarks and road signs. She has to relearn a city and neighborhood that she never left, but which left her behind as it developed around her. They haven't tackled a grocery store yet, but it's on the agenda soon, as well as crossing a bridge so that she can come into my clinic and get to the medical school clinic for appointments.

Standing by has been no easy task. One of the professional practitioners has made a daily phone call to check in. We've covered for each other when we needed to be out of town, but many of my phone calls have been from all over the world. They have had to be short. Calls that give us data and her support, but do not foster dependence. We've had to urge her onto other friends for connection. We had to find that very fine balance between being healthcare practitioners, not best friends.

The medical practitioners involved also ended up supervising a graduate student. Both Cathy and the graduate student will learn lots from the school of "Driving Miss Cathy." Seldom do graduate students have opportunities like this one. Thankfully, there just aren't many examples this extreme. We've had to see Cathy in her home, or in the medical school-clinic close to her home. We've had to shift the boundaries of medicine in this era of HMO insurance and Medicare payments. All of us have had to participate in a labor of love.

Cathy will have to resolve ten years of lost life. We can help with her strength and functioning. We can manage the medications. We can even do additional diagnoses should there be underlying signs and symptoms that persist. We cannot help Cathy resolve her lost life. With her diligence, we are able to help her get well, to get strong, to come back to life. She alone will have to move on through life.

These are the cases where I am left eternally grateful for modern medicine. We have the medications to treat panic disorders. Every year, new medications are made available that are even more specific, more helpful, more effective, and/or have fewer side effects. I often wish that the people in research could see some of these clinical applications up close and personal. I wonder if they know that their dedication gives people back their lives in very real ways. Sometimes, in my frustration about things that don't work, or don't work as well as we want them to, I lose perspective about what we do have that does work. Sometimes, medicine, and our understanding of human physiology, feels to me like we are sitting at the campfire on the tip of the iceberg, and our knowledge is comparable to the tiny amount of ice melted by the fire. Having a Cathy come along allows me to pause. We have come a long way. We can fix some of our mistakes. We all make mistakes. I wish we were more than human, but we aren't.

A story like Cathy's forces me to consider the provocative issues of *quantity* of life versus *quality* of life. The concept of when is someone dead, alive? Or conversely, "When is someone alive, dead?" It forces us to confront the quandary of when, if ever, does society have the right to dictate when to give up, or not to give up or when to allow patients to choose for themselves. I am unconvinced that it is as slippery a slope as many in our society would like us to believe. I think patients are wise. At no time had Cathy given up. Although, as she would laughingly say, there were lots of days that she wished she were dead rather than feel like she did, she never wanted to die. That is a very different picture than patients who are ready and willing to die, but we won't let them.

The right-to-die issue for me is one simply of choice. I do not believe in euthanasia. I will never actively kill someone. I have learned to stand by. There are times, however, when we insist on continuing our intervention to the point that we make dying nearly impossible without struggle. Have we listened carefully to how far patients want interventions to go? Have we stood by patiently, exploring all of the possible options, possible outcomes, and possible points of pause where other decisions can be made? Are we going slowly enough with the information from all of our new technology to allow patients time to adjust to that information? Do we allow choice? These are the ethical questions that belong to practitioners in medicine. The question of when to die is not our question. That one belongs to the patient.

The Gift and Power of Patience
Nicki

Nicki had been an athlete all of her life. A long-distance runner, she was a thin, lithe woman in her mid-forties. She came to me with a wandering injury. I call an elusive injury a wandering injury. It is an injury that has multiple sites of pain or discomfort which seem unrelated. It wanders around the body. One aspect of the injury creates compensations that also cause pain and discomfort and begin to manifest as if they were separate injuries of their own. A medical professional herself, she was baffled by why no one seemed able to make a diagnosis. She was getting worse with everything everyone tried.

It is tough to be a medical professional and become either sick or injured. We certainly don't make the best patients. For the most part, medical professionals aren't patient. We want to understand what is wrong. Unfortunately, left to our own knowledge of what can go wrong, and our own fears, we can make small things big, and big things small. It is tough. When we can't become a "diagnosis," an easy diagnosis, we are easily frustrated and ill at ease.

Athletes don't make the best patients either. Athletes are not very patient. Generally, athletes like being in control, in competition, in good form, and mostly importantly, in good neurochemistry. With good circulation and exercise, the neurotransmitter serotonin increases. Serotonin is a great neurotransmitter. It stimulates and improves the quality of sleep. It improves the quality of muscle relaxation. It serves as our calming, quieting, balancing biochemical. It is our natural anti-depressant. Therefore, when we stimulate all of these qualities with exercise, we feel better. When we are used to this quality of life and it disappears because we cannot exercise at the level we have become accustomed to, we simply do not feel good.

When, in one patient, we combine the qualities of being a medically trained professional and being a well-trained athlete, we usually do not get a great patient. In fact, when an injury brings people with these combinations in their personal history to a screeching halt we end up with patients who are not kind, cooperative, endearing people. Nicki was both medical professional and athlete. She couldn't walk with ease, much less run. She couldn't stand without pain. She couldn't sleep without being awakened by the pain. She couldn't tolerate being in a car going over railroad tracks because the vibration caused pain throughout her entire body. She couldn't lean forward, which she had to do in her work.

When humans cannot stand, sit, or lie down without pain, we are not comfortable enough to be alive. When we cannot walk, run, sleep, or even eat comfortably, we soon lose interest in being alive. When we do not have our own internal chemicals which help define "well-being," we cease to *be* a well being.

A person in this level of discomfort is often partially diagnosed as depressed. Often this leaves the patient feeling their discomfort, which they feel is in their body, is being defined by their physician as "in their head." Depression does not fully describe a person in this level of discomfort. This is more than emotional, it is more than physical. It soon encompasses the realms of emotional, mental, and spiritual. Losing the faith that we can understand what is wrong, no less heal, becomes life-threatening.

I had Nicki move, as limitedly as she could move, through a series of walking strides, attempting to stand on one foot, sit, move from sitting to standing, holding her hand forward while walking, climbing a few stairs, and leaning forward, as if to tie a shoe. All of these movements produced pain. Each of these movements resulted in tension. Every movement pattern was a series of jolts and jerks of movement, not a fluid, flowing movement that a well-oiled human can do with proficiency. I fully understood why her internal medicine physician had thought her injury was a red herring and was masking a neurological problem. Her limitations were so all encompassing, it looked neurological. She had been fully worked up. There were CT scans, MRIs, and electro-stimulation evaluations. Many dollars and much time and medical proficiency had gone into these work-ups. Yet everything was negative.

The next phase of her medical evaluation had been psychiatric. She had been sent for an evaluation of depression, perhaps needing a disability to provide a "time-out" from a very busy practice. The psychiatrist had determined that she was indeed depressed and put her on anti-depressants and sleeping medications. That helped her sleep and her mental status, but did not change her pain or inability to function. The doctors began blaming her, and she cooperated by beginning to blame herself. A referral to a pain clinic produced pain medications. This helped her pain but not her ability to function. She still could not walk, sit, or stand with certainty. Very perplexing, in an academic way. For Nicki, it was flat out terrifying.

As I watched Nicki's jolting, jerking movement patterns, it became clear that she had a failure in a major stabilizing system of her body. We are a very intricate series of levers and leverage. The human form in movement is a study in physics. If we lose a fulcrum, a center from which our movement can stabilize, we cease to move with flow and efficiency. It is like a teeter-totter without a central bar. It simply will not go up or down. A flat board lying on the ground cannot have a flow of action. Nicki had lost the stability in her pelvis.

The sacroiliac joint is the fulcrum for the teeter-totter movements in the human body in all movement planes. All too often it is taken for granted. The three bones which make up the pelvis (ischium, ilium, and pubis) become a moderately "fixed" structure in an adult. We actually rename this fully "grown" bone group the innominate structure. It is then attached to the vertebral spine at the end of the vertebral column at the sacrum. The two parts of the pelvis attach in front at the pubic symphysis. The bones are attached by ligaments. Ligaments attach bones to other bones. They are the guy-wires of the human body. They have many nerve endings because we need the constant feedback of where bones are in relationship to other bones. Unfortunately, they are very avascular (few blood vessels), so they do not heal well if injured.

Women have an additional "good news, bad news" issue with ligaments. The female pelvis is somewhat wider and deeper than the male pelvis. The structure of the female pelvis allows for childbirth. Even with this "deeper bowl," a human child is born when it has to be born in order to get the head through the opening of the mom's pelvis. We are the only mammal on earth born absolutely helpless for a long period of time. If we were born when we were able to hang on to our parents, or run with our herd, we would not be born until the eighteenth month. This thought usually strikes terror in the heart of every female who has given birth, or every male who has watched a birth. Eighteen-month-olds are *way* too large to fit through the opening in the human female pelvis.

Even born as small and as young gestationally as we are, the pelvis still has to stretch. It accomplishes this by a thrust of hormones that affect the pelvic ligaments. The ligaments become quite flaccid. This is what occurs when pregnant moms wake up one day and don't have a leg to stand on, when their balance shifts, when their back hurts, when they waddle like a duck instead of walking like a human. This also may account for the "icky-achy" back of pre-menstrual syndrome (PMS). Any female who has experienced flaccid ligaments can tell a story of the diffuseness of the pain. It is hard to pinpoint an area. There may be one central point of pain, but it is accompanied by a large area of "back ache" that is relentless and ever-changing.

When a ligament in the sacral-iliac group is injured, the pain can be equally diffuse and relentless. Every change in hormones that occurs throughout a month's cycle will bring its own changes in ligament flaccidity along with the injury. This combination helps define why the pain increases and decreases. It also helps explain the changes in function in a sacral-iliac (SI) ligament injury. Nicki had so little stability that standing on one foot was virtually impossible. Her entire body went into a non-rhythmic shaking and she began frantically searching for a wall, another human, or a chair or table to grasp to prevent herself from falling over. The effort to stand on one foot was painful and exhausting. It takes a lot of muscles to shake and move and compensate through-out the entire body. Any time we use that many muscles that inefficiently, we have spent a huge amount of energy doing so. It is not surprising, then, that the body is signaling with any and every alarm system it can to let us know we are at risk.

The human is designed to survive. We are elaborately wired to survive. We are driven to survive. If we were not cleverly and successfully wired for survival, we wouldn't have. Our genetic material for survival would not have been passed on down through the ages. Our pain is our alarm system. We pay attention to pain. We pay more attention to increasing pain or pain that continues over a long duration.

When we hit our arm on the edge of the counter, we usually utter a verbal response . . . "ouch" or something more profane, immediately give ourselves "first-aid" by rubbing the area, and we may even reach for an ice cube to rub on it if it hurts a lot. The ice becomes our local anesthesia, and off we go. A day or so later, we may notice the bruise in the mirror, and wonder where we got it. We may or may not be able to piece the injury back together. It simply wasn't significant enough to hold our attention.

We might wake up one morning, get out of bed, and find a

pain in our body that we didn't have the night before. We usually verbally complain about it, internally or externally, rub it, warm it up in a shower, and if the pain and "stiffness" go away, we ignore it. The body goes through a healing process outside of our awareness. This is efficient.

If, however, the body cannot heal itself with our initial interventions, or the injury actually leaves us vulnerable (we couldn't run-flight, hit-fight, or hide-freeze), our alarm systems continue to go off. The more vulnerable we are, the greater the alarm mechanism. The greater the dysfunction of the body, the greater the inefficiency of the energy expended. The greater the energy expended, the more the alarm systems go off. This is not about pain being out to get us, but rather the pain calling our awareness to our vulnerability. This is our body trying desperately to warn us actively enough that we will proceed with caution and survive.

Nicki and I had a dilemma. I was in favor of getting off the pain medications, listening to the alarm systems, and gradually building the strength of the muscles and tendons surrounding the ligament injury, and rehabilitating the area. Nicki was afraid of the pain. The thought of going off the pain medications brought tears to her eyes and terror to her body. The "what ifs" played in her head as a discordant cord. The kind of symphonic melancholy that places audiences on the edges of their seats, waiting for a violent death scene. She was immobilized by the perception and memory of her unmedicated pain. We struck a compromise. We would start her on a swimming program. As she increased her swimming time, she agreed, reluctantly, to decrease her pain medications.

There are just a few things I like best in the whole world for patients to do. I like oxygen. I like water. I like movement. I like eating real food. If we can accomplish these things, I feel patients can move forward on their own. Breathe deeply. Drink water. Eat appropriately. Move freely. These are my treatment goals. Nicki hurt when she took a deep breath. Nicki associated drinking water with taking pain medications. Nicki could not sit long enough to enjoy eating. Nicki could not move without pain. There was not one treatment goal that did not have to be addressed.

Swimming, being submerged in water, is not only a holy ritual, it is a form of healing. To suspend the pull of gravity on the human surface allows changes in pressure and movement that simply cannot be achieved in gravity. I've hungered to go into space to work on experiments of tissue healing in a weightless environment. Not everyone can tolerate the movement of weightlessness; most people can tolerate water. On this planet, water is as close as we can come to weightlessness. Even people who can't swim can attach an aqua-jog belt and float. Swimming pools are now everywhere. Defining a swimming program for rehabilitation allows patients to take responsibility for themselves. It empowers them to be in control. Some people like to swim in the morning, others during the day, some in the evening. It needs to be something they can put into their own lives.

Rehabilitation takes time. This is a problem for patients attempting to continue to work. I am always thankful when patients have disability insurance and can afford the time to put all of their energy into a healing process. Unfortunately, Nicki had spent a good deal of her disability time in pain, not in process. Now, we had limited time to get to work. We also had an added problem in that she had to be off the narcotic pain medications before she could return to work.

We began. Nicki liked to exercise, but she did not like to swim. *Tough.* She agreed to bite the bullet and at least try it. I asked for ten minutes every day for one week. She complained. It was going to take her longer to get to the pool, undress and redress, than exercise. My experience is to start slow and increase very gradually. Build up in specific ways. The first week, she could not actually swim. She used an aqua-jog belt and gently moved in the water. We had chosen a warm water pool so that she wouldn't get cold. However, it was further from her house. She found that the cool temperature actually made her muscles ache less. The first week behind us, we added one minute per day, per week. At week five, we agreed to add one minute every three days, provided she had no additional pain. This was also the week we agreed to begin reducing her pain medications. On week ten she began to actually swim, crawl and breaststroke with a mask and snorkel so that she did not have to turn her head or worry about the rhythm of breathing. Each week, we also met for one hour of massage, passive and active range of motion, and adaptation to functional skills, like how to get out of a chair. By week twelve, Nicki was getting stronger, sleeping better, and feeling hopeful. My job was cheerleader and coach.

One adaption we had chosen to enable Nicki to walk was to add an elastic/Velcro belt across her hips. This force-loads the joint. The belt became her SI ligament, allowing her to move without having to use muscles throughout her entire body. I believe in this kind of bracing for healing. Many professionals and patients consider this form of assistance to be a crutch, and therefore, to be avoided. I consider this force loading of the SI joint vital to restoring function as quickly as possible. In the case of SI dysfunction, I also feel that force loading the joint allows the ligaments as much opportunity to heal as possible. Sometimes, they will heal, other times there will be some form of permanent injury and corresponding disability. With the belt in place, Nicki could walk. Nicki could stand. Sitting was still out of the question. Bending forward was not possible. There were things in her professional duties that she could do standing up. So, on a limited basis, built around her primary daily activity of swimming, she returned to work. She was not the first physician patient with an SI dysfunction who had returned to work, doing all of her work standing up. I am sure it caught many patients off guard when she took full medical histories standing up, writing on a fully extended hospital tray. Each of these increases in activity allowed her to feel better.

Nicki longed to be able to go out to dinner with her husband. We found there was a window of a few days in each month where she could tolerate sitting for forty-five minutes. Humans are remarkable adapters. Our survival as a species is, in my opinion, about adaptation and denial. Nicki and her husband were no exception. They found that by ordering by phone at their favorite restaurant, they could time their arrival to begin eating. This adaptation was not glorious or romantic, but functional. By adding a bit of diversity and luxury to Nicki's life, it helped both her and her husband to feel less impoverished by her injury.

Families play a vital role in whether or not a patient has enough support to heal. It is much easier to rally behind someone who has a visible injury, a surgery, or an acute illness. It is less easy to continue to pick up the slack day after day for a "non-visual" disability. Pain cannot be flashed on a forehead. Most patients quit reporting pain because it bores them. They don't want to constantly talk about their disability. When someone asks them how they are, they are just as likely as the rest of us to respond by saying, "fine." This is a double-edged sword. Family and friends really want to hear that they are "fine," and immediately presume them to be "better" or at the very least "improving."

Most families are easily able to support for a while, and then resentment begins to build. Usually, resentment builds proportionately to the duration of the disability. After a surgery, when a physician says, "Healing will take six weeks," people mentally, if not physically, mark their calendars and say to themselves, *Good, I will be back to normal by six weeks. I can tolerate anything for six weeks.* It does not occur to them that the reality is that they will heal the tissue for six weeks, and then begin a rehabilitation process that may take them months or years. They then begin the process of learning what adaptations need to be learned to live with the "new, changed me." Sometimes, the healing process goes right on schedule. Six weeks . . . done. Magic. More often than not, however, six weeks is the beginning, not the ending.

Nicki, at six months, was now up to her goal of swimming for thirty minutes. Not swimming each and every day meant pain. She was also walking every day for thirty minutes with her husband. She was off her pain medications and sleeping pills. She was still not fully back to work. She still wore a brace. She was still exhausted, and usually in bed by seven-thirty at night. She was impatient. There were sessions of tears and fears that this was as good as it was going to get. She hated the limitations. She hated that she couldn't garden, cook a meal, or throw a dinner party.

She was well enough to be dangerous. I tread lightly during this period of rehabilitation. This is the point at which, propelled by the combination of desperation and strength, patients can re-injure themselves. It is right at this stage in the healing and re-strengthening process that we have the greatest tension. "I am not going to get any better than this, so why not just do (whatever it is) anyway?" Unfortunately, this generally couples with enough strength and enough resolution of pain to actually go right out and do it.

In Nicki's case, the "it" was to re-stain a deck on her hands and knees. It was summer. The deck needed to be resealed. It was warm and sunny. She was bored with swimming and walking. She felt better. She thought that I was being way too conservative. She needed to prove to herself that she could do it. More often than not, when a patient comes back in, in tears and terror, and almost always shame, I ask why they did their "it." The answer almost always is, "Because I could!" Fortunately, setbacks are just that . . . setbacks. They are not lethal nor irreplaceable.

Over the years, I have learned that all disability requires change. All change happens in four steps. The first step, and I might add, the only step that anyone else can have any participation in, is awareness. It has always been humbling to me to know that all I can do is educate. Beyond that it is up to the patient. The second step of change is catching oneself having just done a behavior and saying to themselves, *I just did it again.* The third step of change is catching oneself in the midst of doing the behavior and saying, *I am doing it again.* The fourth step of change, and the only step where real change occurs, is catching oneself just before the behavior and saying, *What are my choices?* It is at this fourth step of change that our behavior becomes conscious. *What am I doing? Is that what I want to do? What are the risks of doing "it" in this way? Will it hurt me?*

Where we are in the "change process" defines when we are ready to let go of our "crutches," be they braces or canes. This is when we are ready to truly step out "on our own" as fully conscious, participating beings. It is at this stage that we are truly rehabilitated.

Rehabilitation does not mean that we are just like we were before, or are perfect. It means we are conscious of our new "self." We fully embrace our limitations and strengths. We can count on ourselves to set our limits and define our boundaries. In many cases, patients are better at being "aware humans" having had an illness or injury. We are more fully present human beings having had the process of change thrust upon us. In the midst of the process, it is difficult to see this as a prospect.

At the end of eighteen months, Nicki was healed enough to be at work. She still had to attend consciously to her every move. She continued to wear her brace at work, but began the process of experimenting with it off at home. She was still very tired by the day's end. She remained on anti-depressants, select serotonin reuptake inhibitors (SSRIs) to help maintain her mental status, and also for the benefits of muscle relaxation and sleep cycle normalization. Patients are often concerned about being left on anti-depressants by their physicians. Many times, they come in complaining to me that they think their doctor believes the "pain and injury" is all in their head. Why else would they be keeping them on a psycho-tropic medication? These medications are active adjuncts to musculoskeletal problems. Once patients are educated about the benefits of the medications in a wider context and application, they are very willing to remain on the medications for a longer period of time. The SSRIs have fewer side effects for most patients when taken over a longer period of time than most anti-inflammatories or pain medications. These medications actually assist the healing process in the body. They are not just to help patients feel better.

Nicki was now ready to begin the specific strength training portion of her rehabilitation. Some patients choose weight training. Nicki chose yoga. Many people mistakenly think yoga is for old people or does not build strength. I believe yoga is one of the finest specific strength builders available. It maintains length of the muscle tissue while increasing the ability of the muscle to hold against the resistance of the weight of the body. It also trains the body's ability to maintain oxygen in the muscle tissue (aerobic). Yoga allows the circulation to remain full during the exercise period. The muscle tissue does not go fully into an oxygen starved (anaerobic) status. Yoga positions can also be taught specifically enough to build certain muscles. In Nicki's case, we needed to train the muscles surrounding the SI joint and the hip joint. Nicki had permanent damage that would need to be compensated for the rest of her life. These muscles were going to be trained to become her SI joint. In this two-year rehab period Nicki and I had both come to realize that she had a permanent injury. How much disability she would be left with was going to be directly related to her will and discipline around strength building. She was always going to have to maintain this level of strength.

Nicki also made a decision to use sclerosizing therapy. This is an experimental process where saline or dextrose (simple sugar) is injected into the ligament tissue to stimulate an inflammation. As the body inflames in response to the injected fluid, the ligament swells. This swelling provides stability in some people. Each injection series may include a needle stick as many as ten or twelve times. The needles that are used for the SI are long. It is a painful process. What is interesting is that the moment the injections are done and the tissue begins to swell, many patients immediately feel better. They have stability. In some cases, this will last four to six months. For others, it can be longer or shorter amounts of time. Nicki was one of the successful patients with this form of treatment. She was able to do all aspects of her life for the duration of the inflammation. We could not have accomplished what she could accomplish with the injections without the previous attention to strength-building, however. She can keep the injected inflammation for upwards of eight months by using her yoga practice to maintain the inflammation.

Six years have gone by. Nicki is looking forward to semi-retirement in the next few years. She has returned to being a full-time productive professional. She reports being much better with her patients as a result of her own injury. She and her husband can now participate in long bike trips and tours. She plans her life around her daily yoga practice and schedules one full hour seven days a week. She swims only occasionally. Just because she had to do it, never meant she grew to like it. She walks instead of runs, although I must admit that she has run a few competitive five kilometer runs "just because I can." She cannot do a ten-minute head stand in the center of the room, however. She needs to be able to find a visual point of stability in order to accomplish a ten-minute head stand. She says her pelvis still can't figure out being upside down and stable. She still gets injected once or twice a year.

Nicki will always have an injury that she must adapt to and for. Her injury no longer stops her life. She is fully rehabilitated.

Standing on My Head
Kenneth

Kenneth, or Ken, as he preferred to be called, walked stiffly down the hall. I watched through the glass-paned office door. It would never occur to me not to watch someone walk. I have loved to watch animal movement since I was a child. I would spend endless hours in the Nevada desert watching the mustangs walk, run, stand, dust up while rolling on their backs, and groom one another.

As an exercise physiologist, I was taught to be a skilled "watcher" of human movement. I can reduce human movement and gait patterns to the muscles and joints involved in a matter of moments. This wears very thin on those in my family and friend groups who choose to go with me to a basketball game, ballet, or even the mall. As they watch the game, I watch the bodies. I miss entire plays while caught in the fascination of the movement of the shoulder girdle or pelvis as it propels both the human, of gargantuan size, and the ball toward a hoop.

As Ken moved, or didn't move, as was the fact in this case, toward the door, I could write in my mind's eye what was going on in his back. I hadn't seen the referral slip, but I knew this back had already seen a surgeon's knife. I could tell by the compensation patterns that touched all of the muscles of his body that this surgery hadn't worked out the way it might have. I could see, by the lack of efficiency in the movement, that we were going to be working together for some time. Ken was going to have to relearn how to stand, sit, walk, and run again.

In the 1960s, Keppler and Delacato presented a theory of movement training for children whose movement patterns were poorly developed. They even went so far as to suggest that large muscle movement organization was necessary for small muscle movement, like reading, to be efficient. At the time, this was a cutting-edge concept that met with huge amounts of opposition. The medical community was aghast, as it meant believing that muscles and the nerves that stimulated them, were more than tissue to cut through in surgery. The education community also was aghast as it meant that teaching children to read and write had as much to do with muscles and nerves as it had to do with a brain and teaching model. In both communities, this was a concept with far-reaching consequences.

I was a student of exercise and exercise physiology in the midst of these changes. The anatomy and physiology of it all made perfect sense to me, but it was the kinesiology, the study of the actual movement patterns, that made the most sense. We didn't have the biochemical pieces to work with. The neurotransmitters and hormones that would also play a role hadn't even been discovered. My research focused on adults, not children.

Men were returning from the war in Vietnam at the time. In either World War II or Korea, many of these men would not have come back alive. As the MASH units that brought trauma medicine to the front lines were organized in the Korean conflict, modern medicine, with the additional help of the newly discovered antibiotics, managed miracles. We forget that antibiotics as we know them today are only a half a century old. Men with no legs due to buried mines, men with no arms due to the newer, high-powered weaponry, men with steel still lodged in their brains were returned home for rehabilitation.

These men were returning to college campuses, this nation's hallowed halls, with stairs to climb. Access for wheelchairs and crutches became a national crisis. These were men and women who had served their country who now wanted and needed access to the education they had a right to. Never before had this country witnessed such need. These humans were not going to get well and get out of their wheelchairs. These humans were alive, and severely disabled.

I was working and doing research in a college at the time. It seemed like a research project just waiting to happen. How were these men, boys many of them, going to complete their mandatory physical education credits from a wheelchair? I decided it was going to be in a swimming pool. I argued that they should receive all of the possible services that the physical education department could offer them in the form of weight training and retraining for what remained of their bodies. I also decided that this was a great forum to expose non-veteran students to veterans. It was a working lab for movement training.

In this setting, we went to work. If they had the legs to walk on, our job was to figure out a way to teach them to walk. If they had no legs, our job was to teach them how to use their wheelchairs with efficiency, how to "run" in their chairs, how to get in and out of a swimming pool to keep their arm strength up and yet keep their muscles supple and long, not short and constricted, which limited their movement. These were great teaching moments in kinesiology. These were the opportunities of a lifetime to learn and understand. I am forever in debt to these men, who offered what was left of their bodies for my students and me to learn from them. I only hope, all these years later, that we were as useful to them.

Ken was in the right age group to have been a veteran of Vietnam. He wasn't. His back injury was a combination of genetics and work. He had ruptured a disc in his lumbar back, had a surgical "correction" and woke up after the surgery in more pain than before. He had gone through the standard physical therapy protocol with no relief from the pain nor any increase in movement.

A disc in the vertebral column is a fascinating structure. It is a densely structured membrane-covered bag filled with gelatinous goo. It serves as a shock absorber between the bones in the vertebrae. This is no small job, as our vertebrae are designed to move in multiple directions and with a huge amount of force upon them.

The "back bone" is designed to transfer the weight of the head (between eleven and fourteen pounds in the average human) from the top of the spine to the pelvis. The pelvis is the only set of bones with a large enough mass to support the weight. If you think of the human body as similar to the architectural structure of a building, you realize that we, like a standing building, must account for all of the force above use. Unlike a building, we must also move. The whole thing, when you consider the size of a window or doorway "header" (the much larger beam that transfers the forces above it from side to side so we have a window or door to look out of or walk through) is a miracle.

In a vehicle, shock absorbers are in place to absorb the forces of change in one primary direction, up and down, and only to a small extent diagonally, or side to side. They can be springs attached on two ends with a fair amount of rigidity. Compare that to us. Our shock absorbers have to account for shock from multiple directions simultaneously. They cannot be either "fixed" or "rigid," because they would end up limiting our movement in any given direction. This means that our shock absorbers must be fluid and yet contained, must be able to absorb shock in many areas of possible bone-on-bone compression at once, and be able to hold up for years and years of movement, compression, and abuse.

Small wonder then that human vertebral discs are subject to breakdown. As if our own natural activities weren't enough wear and tear, we add football tackles, motorcycles, horseback riding, and a multitude of other additional movement compression actions that we call recreation. It is amazing to me that most discs survive a human lifetime with no injury or apparent breakdown in the form of bone-on-bone compression and pain. Most humans go through an entire lifetime without back pain so extreme that they are willing to undergo surgery for repair.

Most discs don't actually rupture. As the space between the bones diminishes due to compressions, aging in gravity, or injury, the discs are pushed on so hard by the bones that the membrane and its contents ooze into the space beyond the edge of the bone attempting to find space. All too often, this space belongs to a nerve that resides nearby. It is when the disc pushes against the nerve that the pain warning system goes into overdrive.

The pain of a protruding disc is relentless and sharp. There is no position that makes it better or worse. It is simply "worse" all of the time. This is what drives patients to physicians. A disc you can see on a CT scan or MRI. This means there are objective findings that can support a surgical intervention.

The bad news is that less than 50 percent of these surgeries allow the patient to be pain-free after they recover from the surgery. No one knows for sure why. There have been several research projects that have attempted to address these issues.

One research project asked whether the disc was causing the problem at all. The researchers examined many bodies of people who had died of any cause, looking for vertebral protrusions. They then looked back into their medical histories to find out if they had *ever* complained of back pain. The researchers found no correlation at all. In other words, there were as many people with protruding discs who had never reported pain as there were people with reported pain, as there were people with reported pain, and some with surgical interventions. This does not take into account how people feel pain, or report pain, or any of the other myriad of questions that are left unanswered by this research.

Another research project compared people who had disc problems diagnosed in the same way. Some had surgery, others had conservative physical therapy. At the end of six months, using a popular pain and function scale, they attempted to find out who had the best recovery. Approximately the same number in each group was better. Of those who were better in both the surgical and physical therapy groups, they were both about the same amount better. Therefore, no one can really say that one kind of treatment is superior or why.

Ken was one of the surgical questions. He had a definite disc protrusion that had been well-diagnosed. He had surgery done by a fine neurosurgeon at a fine hospital. His post-operative care had been normal and nothing unusual had occurred. His post-operative physical therapy had been routine and well within normal protocols for this type of surgery. Why then, if everything had gone right, was he still in horrible pain? He reported that the pain was worse now then it had been before the surgery. In his reporting of the pain, he had met with physicians who defended the surgery and did not listen carefully to him.

The issue of medical malpractice always raises its ugly head in these circumstances. I always wonder what this might look like if there were no malpractice involved. In this case, I could not see any malpractice. There was only a not-foreseeable surgical outcome. We want to believe that the outcome of anything can be assured. We want to believe that our body will respond just like everyone else's body to a drug, surgery, or therapy. We want to believe that there is control, and that we or the professionals helping us, have it. In fact, we don't have any of this. We don't have guaranteed outcomes. We don't have control over how people's body will respond. We don't have control.

When we do research and talk about outcomes, we are talking about numbers. Numbers are not people. When we report a percentage, we are talking about numbers, not individuals, and the entire spectrum of possibilities that a human can experience. When we give outcomes, we are talking about categories of responses, we are not telling the stories of each of the people.

Numbers don't lie, they just don't tell the truth. Numbers don't tell the story. A person may fall into the numerical category of successful surgery that was predefined to mean a pain rating of four or less on a ten-point scale six weeks after surgery. Or, it may mean a predefined range of motion at 60 percent of normal, six weeks after surgery. In this case, pain may not be rated a variable at all, because it is too variable. It is impossible to know, without looking at the method of measurement, what the numbers do mean. For certain, they are not the stories, regardless of their meaning.

Ken's story was one of post-operative pain and immobility six months after surgery, long after he *should* have been healed. Ken was getting worse, not better. He was now eight months into a pain pattern. Eight months into no sleep. Eight months into his family being at their wits' end with his disability. Eight months without being able to walk, sit, stand, or move with ease. He was eight months into being less a human than he was. He was eight months into lowered self-esteem and self-image. He was eight months into not knowing if he would ever be better. He was way too close to feeling that this process would never end, and if it didn't, he was ready to die.

That was how my first thirty minutes with Ken went. It was a diatribe of anguish and anger. I suggested to him, upon his asking whether I thought he should sue the surgeon, that he did not need the stress of litigation. I doubted that there was any malpractice that would be found. A poor outcome is different than a poorly done surgery. I felt that our focus needed to be on a good future outcome, not looking backward.

The tissue that gets sliced through in lumbar back surgery is an interesting combination of muscle (meat) and fascia (gristle). The muscle is very vascular (full of blood vessels), the fascia is not. Fascia simply does not heal very well. The multifidus muscle is a very complex, gristly muscle mass. Interestingly, the multifidus muscle shares much of its movement potential, by innervation

75

(nerve responses) and by action, with two other muscles, the transversus abdominus, a muscle that wraps the abdomen, our sides and back, and the muscles of the pelvic floor. When one of these muscles is affected, they are all involved. I suspect that surgical intervention so changes the multifidus muscle that the entire abdominal, lumber back and pelvic floor go into a protective pattern so extreme that it limits total movement and creates extreme pain. It is on this theory that I have worked for years in dealing with post operative lumbar back pain.

This complex pattern plus all of the compensation patterns that develop before, during and after the surgery make up one of the sets of people that does poorly after these surgeries. These may also be people who have a very finely tuned pain mechanism. We are just barely understanding the internal biochemistry of pain and pain modulation. It may be in the not-so-distant future that we will be able to do a blood test pre-surgically that will tell us what kind of pain medications we will need specific to that person. This will be based on our "knowing," by what neurotransmitters are in the blood, how much the person will be able to use their own biochemistry (neurotransmitters) for pain control.

Ken left with hope. We have no way of measuring hope in the blood. We therefore have no way of measuring when hope leaves. We can't determine when despair sets in. "*De*" is a Latin prefix meaning *without* coupled with *sperare* meaning Latin verb meaning "to hope." Thus creating the verb "despair" literally meaning *without hope*. We talk of *desperate*, an adjective, describing the human feeling of hopelessness. We do not have the technology of knowing when these feelings change the biochemistry. Perhaps it is the feelings that drive the pain. Not the pain driving the feelings. Perhaps it can go either way.

Ken was ready to launch onto a rehabilitation program. I worked on the muscles I suspected were involved in his pain pattern. Each one reenacted a pain he recognized. The body is very

76

helpful in these ways. It is willing to be discovered and very cooperative in being helped. We finished thirty minutes of discovery. Ken was sent out with a very specific swimming program.

One week later, he was back having never gotten to a pool once. I began my questions. Was there not a pool available to him? No, in fact he belonged to a club with several pools. One of them was a warm water therapy pool with a physical therapist supervisor. Perfect. I began to make notes for follow-up with the P.T. Was the problem time? No, in fact, he was very motivated to get out of pain so would make the time. Then, what was the problem? Ken didn't swim. In fact, he was afraid of the water. Why he hadn't mentioned this a week earlier? I could only guess. Now our problem was to work it out. Aqua jogging was the obvious answer. A belt holds the person above water. The face does not enter the water, and yet we get the body out of gravity, thus reducing the compression on the bones and lengthening the muscles. In many cases of back pain, I actually prefer aqua jogging to swimming as there is no torque required on the spine at all. Breathing in swimming requires either a torquing or hyper extending movement. In swimming for rehab, we usually use a mask and snorkel to solve this problem anyway. The aqua jog belt was not a fix for Ken's fear, however.

Ken and I decided to meet at his club's therapy pool with the physical therapist. We could kill many birds with one stone this way. I could work with him in the water to address the *how* of aqua jogging as well as the *fear* element of the water. Very carefully and close to the side, we worked. Three of us in the water together, until Ken could find enough comfort to work along the side by himself.

The pool changed Ken's pain immediately. He was loath to get out of it, as his pain returned as he climbed up the pool stairs. This information was diagnostic in itself. Muscles and gravity were involved in his pain. He no doubt also had small postoperative adhesions that needed to be addressed. The pool would help with that as well. Strength and elimination of a pain cycle needed to be the first on list to be addressed.

Adhesions are formed for many reasons in the body. The two most common ones are when there is bleeding at a site. In this case, as the blood gains oxygen it becomes very sticky and gelatinous. It will act like glue adhesing one tissue to any surrounding tissues. It then hardens. In that situation, the areas that would have moved independently of one another move together. This causes friction and additional tearing as the tissues move abnormally. The second common cause is in the healing process itself. In soft tissue healing, the body uses collagen, a complex protein that becomes malleable. The body sends in collagen in the density of the soft tissues it is to repair. In areas where there are different types of soft tissue (in the case of the lumbar back surgery, muscles, ligaments, tendons, nerves, blood vessels, fascia) the collagen can get confused. It will arrive in a density to repair tendon at a muscle site. Since tendon moves far less than muscle, the muscle repair is too dense to complete its normal movement pattern. Mother Nature would use movement to help with the delineation of the healing process. Where there is a pre-existing pain pattern that has already reduced the movement at the site, the motions that would help orchestrate the healing don't occur. The net result is short, tight, fibrous scar tissue that tears every time it is forced to move at all. This repetitious tearing is painful.

These complex healing problems are part of what we refer to as a pain cycle. There are multiple reasons for the pain, all of which have to be addressed. From a patient's perspective, they are in pain and they don't really care *why* they are in pain. They just want out of pain. Sometimes, we can buy ourselves some patience with explanation, but most often the pain has to be stopped. With the pain in place it is difficult to address the reasons for the pain.

I referred Ken to a pain clinic for *temporary* pain control. Temporary, because I knew that once the adhesion worked, and the water exercise program were up and going, he would need less and less medication. Temporary also because there would be a need for us to review the pain to help guide our program.

Masking pain is a two-edged sword. We don't want it, but sometimes we need it. I wanted enough of the pain gone that he could sleep, sit, and walk, but not so much of it gone that he could be injuring himself further. We also needed to use pain as a guide for how the program was coming along.

Aqua jogging is boring. I suggested that he find a friend that he could visit with as he worked in the water. With a friend, his willingness to increase the working time in the water increased. Ken was getting better. Now, it was time to use the general strength we had gained and begin to address the strength he needed to build in the very small specific muscles of his torso and pelvis. I chose Yoga.

I work with a pediatric physical therapist who has done physical therapy for years with newborns and very young children with neuro-muscular problems. I convinced her one day to adapt exactly what she did with newborns and one-year-olds to adults. The specific neuromuscular training movements were exactly what the adults with specific muscles to be addressed needed. She agreed. Unfortunately, the way she could move limbs and torsos in newborns was not exactly the same with large adults. She began to modify yoga to accomplish the very specific muscle movement patterns the adults needed to do. She would not have to physically move their much larger, heavier limbs.

Ken's next "torture" was Yoga. Not just any Yoga, but every specific hand-crafted Yoga positions to learn and strengthen very specific muscles and muscle groups. He now had both aqua jogging and Yoga to do. He could accomplish both at his club, but this increased his hours of rehabilitation. Unfortunately, this came right at a time when, because he was in less pain and was stronger, he was working more. Now, time was an issue. We mutually decided that the Yoga would be done at home with his wife. They could at least be finding some time to be together. She actually liked his Yoga work so much she began to come into the Yoga training sessions, too. She had a "once in a while back ache" that disappeared with the exercises. Soon, she decided that she would do the aqua jogging with him as well. The club time turned into their time, together.

A year later, Ken was totally off the pain medications. Short of the twisting activity involved in playing golf, an ultimate goal, he could do nearly anything he wanted to do, and quite a few things around the house which he didn't want to do. Unfortunately, with no excuse, he had to address these issues directly.

It was time he learned to stand on his head. He was shocked! I explained the reason for inverting the body. When the body is upside down, it demands a much more specific range of motion and strength of the very muscles in the low back we were working with. On one's head, you simply cannot use the large leg muscles as part of the back action. On our feet, these large muscles will take over when back muscle fatigue sets in. The large muscles of the thigh, front and back, are key in the action of the back and pelvis. On our head is a great way to isolate them from the action! Ken wasn't sure. He thought maybe this was further than he was willing to go.

We established that he was a bit afraid of standing on his head. I laughed and reminded him how afraid he had been of the water. Compared to that, this wasn't going to be bad at all. His wife was far more ready than he was. I was thankful that he had a partner in this part of the process. The final incentive, however, was his own goal of playing golf again. No head stand, no golf. It was that simple. Unless we could get the final strengthening of the muscles done, his back was never going to hold up to the eighteen holes of twisting that golf requires.

Another year and hours of head stands later, Ken was back playing golf! He started with lessons from a golf pro and buckets of balls at the driving range. It took months before he was up to four holes. We worked up to nine holes by his playing one additional hole each month. Thankfully, the public golf club where he played frequently was willing to bend all of their rules to allow this to occur. In great part, this was due to a very understanding golf pro.

Ken began using a cart, so his energy could be maximized on the actual action of playing, rather than carrying a bag. This also meant he was aqua jogging, doing his Yoga, and playing golf. Time again became a factor. He managed. At the four-year anniversary of his surgery, he played his first eighteen holes of golf.

Now, he plays eighteen holes of golf, carrying his clubs every weekend. He would love to give up the aqua jogging. I won't let him. He would love to give up the Yoga. His wife won't let him. Ken is healed.

Learning to Live Each Moment
Miles

When I first met Miles, he was the head of the rheumatology department of a large health-care organization. He was a wonderful, well-respected physician in the community. He was the kind of physician patients wait as long as necessary, and sometimes too long, to see. He was at the high point of his career. At forty, he was experienced enough to be really great at his profession yet young enough to work hard, supervise residents, run marathons, and live a well-balanced life. On the outside, he had everything going for him.

On the inside, Miles knew something was wrong. He was fatigued. He was fatigued in a way he had never felt fatigue before. Every physician has experienced fatigue. Medical school is in great part a test of fatigue. Tests constructed on themes of: *Can you think on no sleep?* or *Can your hands coordinate having been rudely awakened from their first hour of rest?* For a physician to report fatigue like he has never felt before is indeed a warning signal. This fatigue was also worrisome because nothing seemed to make it better. He had taken extended vacations. He had cut back on his work hours for a month to see if that made a difference. He had gotten extra exercise. He had taken time for extra sleep. He had taken vitamins and minerals. He had tried anti-depressants. His blood work revealed no anemia or other imbalances that might be a factor. The fatigue persisted. Fatigue, like pain, is very subjective. There isn't a way to weigh or measure it apart from the human experiencing it. Had his blood work revealed anemia, the numbers would allow others to externally "know" in the same way a patient internally "knows."

There were two other symptoms that worried Miles. He had always had a bit of asthma. Usually, his bouts of breathing difficulty were triggered by allergies. By keeping the allergies under control, he could prevent the asthma. Even when his asthma flared, using some inhaled bronchiodilators to decrease the inflammatory response and increase the diameter of the bronchial tubes, he could easily deal with the asthma. Now, he had pain in his rib-cage. The pain seemed to stimulate the asthma. The pain made breathing deeply very difficult. As a result, Miles had increasing numbers of "chest colds" and asthma episodes.

He had also been experiencing word retrieval difficulties. I sometimes call these brain spasms. We all experience this as we age. Women experience the loss of nouns as their estrogen levels decrease (women can describe the object, we just can't name it!). The problem with word retrieval problems is that it drives a person to distraction. To not be able to access a word when you know the word (and you know that you know the word), or even used it ten minutes earlier, is alarming. It is also distracting in conversation, much less thinking. It leads a person to wonder if they are experiencing some form of early senile dementia. Could it be the early onset of Alzheimer's disease? Or worse yet, a series of small strokes? Since none of these possible diagnoses are diseases we want to embrace, people usually aren't anxious to communicate these symptoms out loud.

After dealing with his symptoms in silence for nearly a year, Miles decided that he had to seek further medical evaluation, that went further than blood work, additional rest, and reduced stress at work. At this point, his chest pain had increased and had extended into his left shoulder. He worried that he was having a series of slight heart attacks, as heart problems can also present this way.

Pain is a wonderful motivator. Humans will ignore a lot of

pain. Humans will justify, rationalize, and deny huge amounts of pain. Every human has a breaking point where the pain so intrudes on their everyday existence that they seek help. We seldom die of the pain; we just wish we would. Pain was the final force that drove Miles to return to a physician. He needed his arm and shoulder to accomplish the work he did. He had to have accuracy in his range of motion to accomplish the movements and touch that were a vital part of his everyday work experience.

Unfortunately, everything that Miles was experiencing was a symptom. He had to convince the physician that there was something amiss. Perhaps the threat of not being taken seriously was, in great part, why he waited so long before he sought help. Once the initial blood work was negative, he waited until he had his own arsenal of what made it better, what made it worse, what he had tried in self-management and self-treat options before approaching the fortress of medical diagnosis.

A CT scan showed nothing. Four additional months went by, then Miles, himself insisted on an MRI for a closer, more complete look. An MRI is a costly piece of medical diagnosis. Aside from the thousand or so dollars it takes to have one done, it is also not a pleasant experience. A person is placed on a very narrow, mechanically driven platform, and then slid into a narrow tube. There is air flow, but that is the only redeeming feature. Otherwise, it closely resembles being in a very narrow lava tube while simultaneously being inside a broken washing machine. When "on," the tube rumbles, whines, clanks, and shakes. It could qualify as a carnival ride, but when a person is not feeling well, it is not an experience most people race to have. There are new MRI machines now becoming more available that are far less confining, so as technology moves forward perhaps the negative experience will lessen. At the time, this was done for Miles, however. It was not a way any human being in their right mind would choose to spend an hour or more of their time.

The MRI showed multiple white spots on Miles' brain. Something was certainly wrong. More diagnosis was now necessary. Back to the MRI tube Miles went again. The brain had been exposed, now it was time for his cervical spinal cord. More white spots. A neurologist was called in. A third MRI for a thoracic spinal cord evaluation was ordered. Three MRIs in one week is just about beyond human tolerance, unless of course the person enjoys spelunking. The neurologist was, by this time, quite sure Miles had Multiple Sclerosis. MS is less common in men than women, but not uncommon. Miles was in the right age group and his diffuse symptoms certainly fit the MS pattern. A spinal tap was done to confirm the diagnosis. Unfortunately, MS is not a straightforward disease. The diagnosis for MS is also not straightforward. There are many false negatives from lab evaluations of spinal fluid. The disease is complex, and so is the diagnosis. Very often, it is a combination of tools, patient history and experience that are utilized to actually make an MS diagnosis.

Prior to our new diagnostic imaging tools, MS was a disease that wasn't "seen" in its earliest stages. It wasn't until a patient was into serious degeneration that we were able to establish a diagnosis. Further, there wasn't anything that could be done for the patient, so having an early diagnosis was not useful. There was a period of time, I call it the dark ages of modern medicine, or the era of delusion, when we kept diagnosis and information from the patient. Often we told the families the patient had cancer or MS but wouldn't tell the patient.

This led to some of the most disconnected experiences I've ever seen. The patient would know something was terribly wrong, but everyone around them would carry on as if there wasn't . . . except for the times when the families couldn't hold up under the pressure of it all and would fall apart, leaving the patient wondering what happened or what they had done to create such a reaction.

The only thing that is predictable about MS is its unpredictability. The symptoms of MS will vary from patient to patient and within one patient. Some of the symptoms that can manifest are truly bizarre. Patients report sensory manifestations of mice or shrews running up and down their arms and legs. Never rats. Rats would be much heavier than the tiny feet they experience. Some times the mice and shrews only run around at night, other times they run around after exercise, or while people are attempting to concentrate, but at no other time.

Some patients experience loss of convergent vision, or vision in one eye. Sometimes it lasts forever, other times it is recovered in a month or two. An eyelid may twitch and torque across the eye, and although they believe their vision is impaired, it is the eyelid's loss of muscle control causing the disruption in vision. Sometimes, patients see lightning flashes across their field of vision. Other times, when they close their eyes to sleep, they get a visual field of a broad starry night. Phosphatines as they are medically called. Starry, starry nights of bright stars, some of which fall or become comet-like.

MS can be predominately sensory changes, or it can be loss of muscle control or a combination of both. Pain can be present in MS patients. Other MS patients have no pain whatsoever, in fact, they have large patches of no feeling at all. Some MS patients have fatigue and that is all. Other MS patients have no fatigue, but they have ever-continuing losses in muscle strength and function, finding themselves in a wheelchair in quite short order. There is simply no way to predict for a patient what their experience of this disease will be. The best we can do is to stand by and watch their disease patterns develop. Nowadays, there is a large spectrum of drugs that can be utilized to slow the degeneration, as well as relieve the symptoms. Knowing you have the disease really can help patients to understand what they are experiencing and why. It also allows us to move forward to slow the progression of this disease we have no cure for, yet.

Miles was experiencing too much pain and disability in his shoulder to continue to work. He took a medical disability and left his practice. He tried all the various forms of medications to slow the disease, and found that each of them made him sicker than he was already feeling. His nerve pain was treated with a pain medication designed for nerve pain, and a muscle relaxant. Although some of his symptoms were reduced, he was still feeling very fatigued and far away from the man he had been. I suggested a stringent daily exercise program and ice. We chose swimming in a cold water pool. MS responds best to cool temperatures, although becoming too chilled also increases the muscle spasm. As Miles began a regular swimming program, his muscles lengthened and his fatigue and muscle spasms lifted, somewhat.

Ice for injury, and in this case a disease, provides a true love-hate relationship of a treatment. Putting an ice cube directly on the skin and rubbing or massaging with it is not a romantic experience. It does accomplish miracles, though. Ice does three important things. It is an anesthesia after about thirty seconds. It increases deep circulation, thus improving the amount of blood flow and oxygen to deep muscle tissue. It tricks the body into believing frostbite is about to set in. Frostbite or freezing tissue causes the body to go into a defense position. The body presumes tissue death, so goes about setting up a parameter of its own anti-inflammatory chemicals (cortisone) around the affected area. This gives the body a local hit of anti-inflammatory chemical at the needed site. Icing an area directly only takes about ninety seconds and can be repeated when needed. For MS patients, ice is how many get through a rough day or night.

Ice may be the remedy that allows patients to keep working, or prepare a meal for their family. In fact, there are now ice vests that are designed to allow MS patients to maintain walking, running, or general living. Ice vests free up the hands while keeping an

87

application of coolness going. If they were to do these activities without an ice vest, their body temperatures would go up and their symptoms with it. Since Miles had chosen his extended vacations in warm, sunny areas of the world, perhaps this accounted for his symptoms never decreasing with more rest.

Miles' wife had left him in the midst of the depth of his disease. She simply could not handle the fact that she couldn't reach out to touch him or brush up against him. It hurt. She could not tolerate that he couldn't help out at home, he was in bed, exhausted. She could not reconcile herself to the considerable cut in his income. She became frustrated that his needs were the driving force of their lives: where they went, how long they could stay, where they could vacation were all set by how he felt. She was looking into a very dark tunnel of degenerative disease, and could not see any light, or the end. She was overwhelmed. Although it is sad, divorce is not an unusual experience in degenerative disease. It is very tough on the patient, as it drives home their own losses and sadness. It also leaves them alone, facing losses so profound that they cannot even think about how their life will look down the road, around the corners, at the end. Sometimes, family members are the people who cannot adapt.

Miles began feeling better with ice and swimming. He also began a yoga program to lengthen his muscles. He worked on relaxation techniques. He sold his house, which required a great deal of gardening, and chose instead a small, one-story home that could easily be adapted for a wheelchair should it become necessary. He put in a hot tub for soaking. I guess it should be called a cool tub, as it only exceeded normal body temperature by one degree. He didn't have hoards of friends hoping for invitations to soak. Since he loved to garden, he planned an easy-care garden with beds in elevated planters that he could garden in while sitting in a chair. His new house sat on a hill with a wonderful panorama of the surrounding hills so he felt open in his perspective, while his world was closing around him.

Miles was adapting to his disease in many of the same ways that we all will have to adapt to aging. His choices were not a great deal different than many of the changes that have to take place in a home when joints won't move as easily as they once did.

Miles also decided to return to work as he began to feel more in control of his life. The question was what was it he could do that would make him feel productive and useful, but not be so involved that he would not be able to "keep up." Some jobs lend themselves to scaling back. Limitations can be set by limiting the number of hours spent at work, or changing the nature of how work is accomplished. Perhaps work can be done by computer at home, where a patient can lie down to rest or take a nap midway through the work. Unfortunately, medicine doesn't fit so easily into this mold. Once patients are scheduled, it is hard on everyone if the physician simply cannot work that day, or is unpredictable. When patients expect a physician to be responsive to their needs, it is tough to also be responsive to their own. Miles had to figure out how to make his work fit his disease. After much thought, we all hit upon the possibility of his being a consultant for the student health service at a local university. This allowed him to do much of his work from home, by phone. It allowed him to set the day and time that he could come to the clinic. He could limit his contact with patients to one or two visits, while another physician would follow the patients through a crisis or emergency. This was a match made in heaven. The student health center got a primo physician, that under ordinary circumstances they could not have afforded. Miles got control over a limited work environment.

Where there is a will, there is a way! This was my grandmother's favorite saying. I grew up with it. I tired of her saying it, especially when, as a child, I didn't want to *find* a way! She was right. Adaptation takes will. Miles is about to be married to a woman who sees so many wonderful qualities in him that she doesn't mind the possible limitations. Since there is no way to know if he will get worse, or how or when, she chooses to live in the present. She is a nurse and is not afraid of the increasing disability, should it happen.

Change happens. It can happen to any of us at any time. Living every day in the moment is good practice for all of us, all of the time.

The Gift of Aging and Adaptation
Mildred

Mildred was eighty-two when she walked into the clinic. She came with a walker and a daughter for support. She was referred by a surgeon who had replaced her hip only six weeks earlier. This joined the artificial knee on the other leg. The surgeon's referral note had read that her gait was off and she needed some balance work and strength-building. Simply looking at the bent over figure entering the doorway, anyone would have agreed with his assessment. It was, however, not the whole story.

We ask a new patient to fill out a history card—a written history. This written history opens the window into the patient, a way to know where to begin with our questions of patients. We also take oral histories so that we can learn more about what patients wrote down. Oral histories give us a chance to open the window wider. Oral histories allow us to probe the memory depths and follow up with questions that lead us to other perspectives, or data. We do physical examinations to add information to the written and oral history. This is our opportunity to review the patients and their body from our perspective. This is where we get to see if what we find with our knowledge, palpation, and senses matches with how the patient's story sounds. In a good intake visit, the written, oral, and physical findings are consistent. They build upon one another. There are few surprises. When this is not the case, we, the patient and practitioner, begin our journey with discrepancy. There is not integrity between what was reported and what was found.

Mildred was covered in bruises. There was not one mention of the bruises in her written or oral history. Was this a case of elder abuse? Had she fallen? Did she have so little balance that she reeled from wall to wall even with a walker? Were the bruises there, but failing eyesight did not allow her to witness them herself . . . out of sight, out of mind? What on earth accounted for the bruises? What on earth accounted for not having accounted for the bruises?

A practitioner always has to figure out how to approach a possibly sensitive area. There is very little training spent in medicine on how to elicit information from patients on hard subjects. Somehow, this precious information is supposed to pop into our heads in the moment of need. Ample opportunity exists for blunders and bloopers in medicine. This had the full potential for both. I am not known for tactfulness. I feel the most comfortable with direct communication. Yet, here in front of me, was a woman from another generation, where direct communication was not common and in many cases even unacceptable.

I voted in favor of my hands and not my mouth or brain in this instance. As I scanned her arms and legs with my hands I asked if this area or that area hurt. After asking what seemed to me to be at least one hundred times, Mildred asked why I was asking if she hurt. I explained to her that there were bruises at most of the areas that I had inquired about. "Oh that," she said with a long sigh. "I keep falling." That was the end of her immediate response. I had to take the lead on follow-up questions to try to learn why she was falling. Had she fallen before or after her surgeon had seen her? Had she fallen with or without the walker? Had she fallen multiple times, or just once and in attempting to get up? There were so many other pieces to learn. Mildred was not a story-teller.

Thousands of questions later, I was able to piece together a very scattered and sad story. Her knee replacement surgery had taken place three years earlier. At that time, she and her husband were still living alone in their family home on a lake in a rural setting. After she returned from the hospital, they, with the help of a neighbor, had managed to set up a bedroom for her in the formal dining room, as all of the bedrooms were upstairs. There was a small bathroom on the first floor but it only consisted of a toilet and washbasin.

Together, she and her husband of sixty-two years had managed her post-operative care, her baths, their meals, and the upkeep of the house. He had been a professional, so many of these tasks were in her domain. It was unclear as she relayed the tale who had the hardest adaptation. He had to learn new tasks. She had to give up her work and deal with his imperfection at doing her tasks. As he became more competent at his "new jobs," she had to watch her loss of jobs. Her loss of "jobs" faced her with "retirement." It had never occurred to her, as a housewife, that she too would or could face retirement.

I believe that in relationships with others we create our roles, rules, and rituals. Often these are created unconsciously. Many times, they are established long before a relationship, in our families of origin. We merely slide into the patterns we were taught to hold as children. These are the areas where we feel confident. The areas of our skill, knowledge, and experience, the areas of our personal reward. The roles, rules, and rituals are often forced to change in the midst of injury, illness, pain and certainly aging. The best we can hope for is communication that allows us to acknowledge the change and our feelings about the changes. Sometimes, it is a relief to have adult children step up to the plate and hold the large family gatherings at their house. Other times, this same shift poses a loss, and is filled with grief and anger. Often, this is perceived to be a temporary change, and the displaced role or ritual can be reestablished when health returns. All of these things are possible if there is communication. Unfortunately, as often as not, there is no communication. There is not even awareness of the dynamic that is occurring. These social issues play very specifically into health, these are aspects of life that should be part of the medical providers domain. Seldom is there time any longer to identify these issues, much less address them.

Mildred was her husband's burden and she felt badly about that role; so badly that she had pushed herself, by her own admission, to exhaustion. Beyond exhaustion. Wanting so badly to be better, to be back to her "old self," to relieve her husband of his growing list of tasks, she had pushed until she was barely able to move by the end of each day.

I spent a lot of time wondering why there had been no medical social worker on this case. Why had there not been a home health care assessment? Had they both been too proud to accept one? Had those forms of intervention not been offered? If not, why not? How had these two people with good insurance, highly educated, very capable under normal circumstances, slipped through the cracks of good medicine?

Six weeks to the day after her surgery, the day she was to return to her surgeon for her last appointment, her husband dropped to the floor, with a stroke. He emerged from a coma three days later completely paralyzed on his left side and unable to speak. It was her turn to nurse him. They returned home four weeks later, where she became his primary-care provider.

I have seen stories like this one all too often. Without the proper support services, resources, and respite care the caregiver gives out before the care that needed to be given is completed. Sadly, this couple, like so many others, had not taken care of business. They had not worked on issues like giving up a family home. Their beautiful home, filled with memories, was too large to easily care for. A smaller home surrounded by family and friends who were easily accessible would have been a much better option. Creating space for that transition before either of them were ill would have been a blessing. Change is hard, and fear of change is often paralyzing. To make those changes would have required acknowledging the life changes in themselves.

They had not taken care of trusts or wills. They had not dealt with financial issues, learning the tasks of decision making, check-writing, credit cards, bill paying. So many women my age take all of these tasks for granted, but many women have never paid a bill or written a check, or invested in or sold stock. "His" and "her" jobs were divided along the lines of expertise and interest, if not political and social norms.

It had never occurred to them what would happen if the person behind those jobs couldn't do them. They had not spoken openly about the end of their lives. They had not considered aloud with each other what was acceptable care or intervention. They had not walked the path of life's end. We find ourselves in this dilemma frequently. Death used to be something we could speak openly about simply because it happened. Now, it is hidden.

Immediately after the death of her husband, Mildred's children decided it was time for her to sell the family house. Mildred had children living in various locations all over the United States. They felt that Mildred needed to move into one of their homes for her own safety. The family home was sold. Mildred was moved with a few of the family belongings across the United States. Mildred had lost her support mechanism and familiar surroundings. Normally, I don't use other aspects of life as a metaphor, but in this case, it just seemed too obvious. Mildred fell. Mildred fell and fell. Mildred had lost her support systems, she didn't have a sense of balance or stride. She had lost everything that was familiar to her.

Mildred needed to get her sense of self back before we could work on her balance. She needed to want to stand up and see the world before we could work on her gait. Mildred had to want to live before we could help her build strength. There were real issues. Mildred had choices to make.

Mildred did not want to live with her daughter, son-in-law, and grandchildren. Frankly, there was too much commotion and

change in surroundings. Every day found toys, clothes, and posses-
sions in different places than where she had encountered them
before. She would wake up during the night and not remember
how to move herself through the tangled web of her room to the
bathroom down a hallway. She had too many things for her one
small room, but she did not want to give up one more aspect of
herself. These things represented the final threads of the well-worn
cloak of her life.

Mildred did not know how to ask for what she wanted. She
wanted to find a small house and attempt to live independently.
She actually wanted to go home but didn't dare raise her hopes that
high. She felt her family had made decisions based on her well-
being, not on her *being well*. She was afraid she would offend them.
The more questions I asked, the more complete the story became.
Mildred was lost. She was lost *inside* herself and *outside* herself.
Rehabilitating people against their will is not possible. There is no
mechanism that we can force on patients that rehabilitates them
without their being present for the experience.

Mildred explored the possibility of hiring a companion during the day to help with cooking, cleaning, and even dressing herself. She was now thinking of giving up her "work" to a stranger,
not to her husband, as had happened before. She contemplated
driving again, only to realize she didn't even know the area in
which she was living. There were no familiar landmarks to help
guide her. She had come to the area worn out and worn down. Displacement is frightening at any age. The feelings of vulnerability
and desperation seep in along the edges of our boundaries of self
until we can not sort out where our environment begins and our
self ends. She was in new territory, with no vistas to help sort it out.

One day, while taking a walk down the hallway outside our
office, she remarked that she had finally learned the hall, and as
long as no one opened an office doorway suddenly, she felt safe. A
hallway that she had walked hundreds of times as we worked on

gait and posture. She finally felt safe in a *hallway*. Could this woman ever walk by herself on a sidewalk?

Sidewalks are made for humans with good feet, balance, neuromuscular control, and eyesight. With the addition of the new cutaway curbs, they are also made for motorized wheelchairs and carts. They are not designed for anything or anybody in between. Cracks, uneven surfaces, protrusions, parking meters, bike racks, bustling hustling people, garbage, sidewalk café chairs and tables are all things we, the sighted and able bodied take for granted on a sidewalk. We know how to access and walk around. Those who can't see to make the accessment or move with ease around these impediments find them true stumbling blocks.

Heavy doors keep out the cold wind. Heavy doors also keep out those who do not have the strength or balance to pull or push them open. Every business that wants people to enter its domain should ask someone with physical disabilities to try their business out. The blind can find assistance from a seeing eye dog. The people with neuromuscular disabilities, strength, or balance dysfunction can't use a "be your muscle" dog. We as a society severely limit access without even realizing it.

Mildred needed to begin some strength-building work. Her hip replacement had been set at an angle slightly off her center of gravity. This may have been a calculation error, a limitation caused by the nature of her own bone and how the prosthesis fit into the bone tube, or it could have been slippage that happened as the glue agent set up. In any case, she would have to learn to compensate for the angle displacement. A warm water swimming pool would certainly be the best solution. Out of gravity, we could increase the range of motion of the surrounding joints, and begin the strengthening work of her entire body.

Access to resources poses problems of money, transportation, mobility, supervision, and time. For Mildred, time was not an issue. Finances were. Transportation and mobility certainly were.

97

She was a five-minute taxi ride from her home to a high school pool that had public swim hours, but as it was used primarily for high school competitive sports, the temperature of the water made it impossible for Mildred's thin body. Her water time would be limited by the hypothermic factor. She would be too cold.

A warm water pool with supervision by a physical therapist for physical disabilities was also close by. Additional taxi fare would be off set to some degree, as her insurance would pay some of the cost of the program. She was deeply stressed as it was run by the Jewish Community Center and she, a devout Catholic, was unsure she would feel welcome. As we explored this further, she was unsure she would feel comfortable interacting with Jews. Here, we were faced with limitations we seldom recognize in medicine . . . a political/social blockade to treatment.

After a great deal of pushing, along with the recognizing that her alternatives were a much greater distance and cost away, she agreed to try the JCC program. What happened next was a miracle. Not only was she welcome, she was embraced. In the group of elderly men and women, she found companionship. There were hip and knee replacement stories to be told by nearly everyone in the pool, a few cardiac stories, but mostly orthopedic stories. There were hearts and hands that needed holding and touching, just like hers. There were people who had not been uprooted from their cities, but were just as uprooted in their "home town" by having to move into a retirement community for care and supervision. There were many walkers and canes "parked" along the pool's edge. There was coffee and tea and sandwiches at the snack bar to be shared. There were invitations to bridge games and wine-tasting gatherings. There was community.

Mildred had found a home in the pool. The physical therapist and I laughed one day as we visited by phone, because our problem was that she talked so much there wasn't a lot of exercise going on. We decided to move her to a deep water aqua jog program, so at least while she talked, she had to keep moving.

Mildred flourished. With support from her new friends who had lived in the city, she was able to find a small house on one level, with a small garden to tend. The house was close to public transportation, and others in the "pool program" (the Pool Club as we soon began to call it) who could help with transportation. She also became part of a telephone tree. The Pool Club members checked up on each other morning and night by telephone. Religious and ethnic barriers melted down to nothing. Kindness prevailed.

A year later, a car, after her driver's license was reissued, she had crops of garden flowers, and multiple visits from her kids who stayed in her extra bedroom and cooked with her in her own kitchen, Mildred fell again. In the eighty-year-old age group, we cannot be quite so cavalier about setbacks. Thankfully, she had no broken bones, but the amount and degree of soft tissue damage was stunning. Worst of all, the amount of open skin lesions required her to be away from the Pool Club. The community held together, but the gains in strength and self-esteem began falling away quickly.

In the elderly, and in those with degenerative disease processes, losing time in a strength program can be life threatening. For Mildred, it was. She began to have serious edema (swelling) problems. The water had helped with circulation and dehydrating her tissues, so we simply had not seen the edema. Now, it was there in extremes that were frightening. We began a full work-up. We looked at heart function, kidney function, and chemistry problems. At the end of too many doctors, we discovered that Mildred was well into a complete kidney failure. This time, her falling was not about strength or gait. Her falling was about the end of her life.

Mildred, with her children gathered around, discussed all of the options. A physician family member wanted her to begin dialysis. Mildred said no. The thought of being hooked up to a machine three or four times a week, of not being able to be in the pool, of losing that level of independence again, was more than she was willing to do. At nearly ninety, she was ready to call it quits.

Mildred took care of business. She met with her internal medicine physician and spoke about how she wanted comfort levels to look. She hired a round-the-clock nursing service, interviewing the caregivers herself. She marked all of her belongings, had a party with her Pool Club members, signed that final mass of legal papers, and then went to bed.

Mildred's family was upset that Mildred had hired around-the-clock nursing service. They felt among them they could do the caretaking. Mildred held firm. She announced that she wanted them to be there to support her emotionally, not be burdened by her physically. She also explained to them that she wanted to maintain her privacy and dignity in relationship to her children and grandchildren. She did not want them "cleaning her up." I was pleased that they honored her wishes. Her death was able to happen quite simply, as she had planned it.

A week later, Mildred was dead. Her wishes were that her body be taken back to her home town and be buried next to her husband. The entire family flew back with her remains and held the funeral on that same day. A perfect ending for a perfect lady.

Learning Beginnings and Endings
Johnathan

Johnathan was a thirteen-year-old patient with leukemia in the days before the breakthrough technologies of bone marrow and stem cell transplants. Johnathan had survived two rounds of chemotherapy with all of the side effects of the drugs in that era of chemotherapy drugs. Nothing had worked. The cancer cells continued to grow.

Cancer is an interesting disease. Cancer is a part of us. It is not an external event in time and space. It is not something from outside of ourselves that invades our being. It is us, our own cells, growing without appropriate differentiation or proper messages to slow down or stop.

Cancer was named after the sign of the ancient zodiac calendar. The Latin word *zodiac* means round. The Greek *zoidiakos* translates into circle, and *zoidion*, as animal. *Cancri* is the Latin translation of the Greek word *karkinos* meaning crab, thus, the sign of the crab. Calling the disease cancer is due to early observations of dead humans. As people who had died of cancer were prepared for burial, cancerous cell growth looked like a large tumorous area with projections that looked like crab legs extending from the body of the crab. All cancer received its name from these ancient observations. Not all cancers look like a crab in the human body, as is the case with leukemia. Without microscopes and our modern ability to see, the ancient observers could only name what they could see with the human eye.

Johnathan did not look like a crab. In fact, for the most part,

Johnathan did not look or act like a sick kid. Unless you could watch him day in and day out, you would not have guessed that Johnathan was ill at all. Instead of growing each day like boys in this age group are not only prone, but obligated to do, Johnathan shrunk. Part of his shrinking was due to the effects and side effects of the chemotherapy. He wasn't very hungry. He had a haircut that looked more like a shave, giving his head a smaller than normal look. He was very thin. Beyond his looks, however, Johnathan was a thirteen-year-old boy, through and through.

Johnathan was a nursing nightmare. He lived in a skilled-care facility with sixty-five other patients, most of whom were much older. Children do illness and death far differently than their adult counterparts. They live until they die. Adults spend a great deal of their final "living time" dying. Johnathan would have none of it. He knew he was dying and was not at all reluctant to talk about it, but on the other hand, if there was living to do, he was involved in it.

He would pour lemonade under the wheelchair of a sleeping wheelchair-bound patient. Assuming the patient had an "accident," the nursing staff would immediately go into a clean-up mode, awakening the sleeping patient for a clothing change and floor wipe, only to find that they'd been had. Red Jell-O in a urine bag had much the same effect. Assuming urinary tract bleeding had begun, the patient would be "worked up" for serious urinary problems only to find that Johnathan had struck again. When he could commandeer a vacant wheelchair he would turn any hall into a race track, putting people and things in immediate danger of being "road kill." He would force the entire staff to laugh as he made faces that matched exactly the faces of the other residents. He would tell jokes, stand on his head and entertain those needing to be entertained, whether they wanted to be entertained or not. He was a delight and a pain in the ass, continuously and simultaneously.

I was working two days of day shifts, two days of swings, two days of graves and then having two days off. As a result, I didn't know my name, much less what day it was. On this particular Tuesday, I arrived back at work beginning my next round of days. A Monday on a Tuesday. A day shift in daylight.

I stuck my head into Johnathan's room to say hi. I found him with his feet propped on his pillows, his head at the foot of the bed, and his body loosely tied in restraints.

"Oh dear," I said. "Not a good morning, already, huh?"

"Nope," he responded, "too much salt in the sugar bowls at breakfast."

I began the educational lecture that we'd had so many times before about how people on salt-restricted diets really couldn't have those kind of pranks pulled on them. Once again, we went through the discussion of it wasn't just about how it made their coffee taste, or to determine if they could still taste and spit. Watching the response of "proper old ladies" (usually wearing wigs from cancer-caused baldness) both spit and lose their wigs, was exactly the impropriety Johnathan was looking for. For this early morning coffee chaos, Johnathan was on "bed-tied time out."

As I edged to the door to take my leave, Johnathan asked me whether I was working Saturday night. I began my finger count-off of my schedule.

"Well, I have two days of days, that's today and Wednesday, two days of swings, that would be Thursday and Friday, and so, Saturday, I'll start my first day of graves. Why?" I asked.

"What time do you come in to work then, on Saturday?" he responded.

"I usually get here between ten thirty and ten forty-five, report is at eleven," I answered.

"Would you come in a little early that night?" Johnathan asked, looking back over his forehead at me, standing at the doorway behind him. He had an elf-like grin on his face, and I feared then and there that I was about to become a player in one of Johnathan's one-act pranks.

"I usually don't hang around here without pay," I responded, "I like the place, but not that much." I asked again the question, "Why?"

He said, quite matter-of-factly, "Well, Sue, that's the night I am going to die and I would like you to be here to hold me in the rocker."

I was so astonished that I must have stood there with my mouth wide open. Johnathan himself broke the silence.

"What's wrong with that, Sue?" he said. "I should be able to ask for what I want, right?"

Having now had a moment to recover, I asked him how he had arrived at Saturday night. Johnathan responded without a moment of hesitation.

"Well, I've been thinking a lot about it. I want to watch the Red Sox play on Saturday and the game is at two. Sunday is my sister's birthday so that will give my mom and dad something to be happy about. I think it is the right thing to do."

It never occurred to me to ask him *how* he knew he would die on schedule or *how* he was going to make sure that it happened the way he wanted it to. I went for the question of my own comfort.

"Why do you want me to hold you?" I asked. "Don't you think that is a job that your parents should do?"

"They will be too sad to do it right," he said in a matter-of-fact tone.

"How do you hold someone right?" I asked.

"Well," he replied thoughtfully, "you hold them tightly to you, like a baby, and rock the chair all the time until they quit breathing.

You might even hum or sing, if you think of it."

"Or if I can!" I said.

"What do you mean, Sue?" he responded. "You hum and sing and whistle around here all of the time. That's how I know you're coming!"

I now knew why I had never caught the little bugger in the midst of any of his pranks!

"I wasn't thinking of 'if I can' in the sense of, can I sing or hum or whistle?" I said. "I was thinking of it in the sense of *will I be able to* hum or sing or whistle. I will be so sad that I would cry or want to cry. It's just a bit tough to hum or sing or whistle if you're crying."

"Why would you cry?" he said, now turning his face slightly to the left to look more directly at me as I had edged back into the room. "If I want to die, and I've planned to die, why would you cry? I don't get it."

This is the kind of question about death only a child would ask. They haven't had the years of social brainwashing about death and what is proper etiquette surrounding death. Every child I have ever worked with who was in a dying process took death in stride. It was expected and they could reflect on death from a multitude of tangents, all of which made perfect sense to them, and almost no sense to the adults.

In the same way that it would not have occurred to me *not* to cry, it had not occurred to Johnathan that I *would* cry. In fact, from his perspective, since he had planned the party, thoughtfully giving consideration to everyone involved, we should all be there to celebrate. I am not sure it would have occurred to his parents that they should be glad at his sister's birthday the next day, any more than it would have occurred to Johnathan that his sister's birthday would be forever changed.

I called the social worker and suggested that we have a visit with Johnathan's family, and check the schedule for the Red Sox game, as if I wasn't sure he was going to be absolutely correct about the schedule and time. We all met and then met with Johnathan. He was just as matter-of-fact about the whole process with all of us as he had been in our initial conversation. I also have to admit that we did not give his timetable much credence. We all *know* that we don't just plan our death down to the day and hour a week in advance.

The staff decided to go about their business. We all paid a little more attention to Johnathan, checking his vital signs a bit more closely, and keeping track of items that might be used in a suicide attempt. There was no change in Johnathan to speak of. He was his usual prankish self.

The week wore on. It was a hard week in many other ways. A couple of other patients died. A few others were readmitted to the hospital. A staff member quit. All of our attention was not focused on Johnathan. By Friday night, I was tired out, and I still had two nights of graveyard shift to go. As I left work, after report at nearly midnight on Friday, I left a note to call me if any change in Johnathan occurred. I also told them I'd call in if I was going to be away from my phone. I was not planning on being away from my phone, but I was worried that I was so tired I'd sleep through a call!

I awoke around ten in the morning. I called in first thing, only to find out that Johnathan was on restrained bed rest for wheeling over the foot of one of the nurses. I requested that his "bed-tied time out" end by two so that he could be upright for the game. With great reluctance, the weekend day-shift agreed.

Weekend staffs run lean. There are as few people as possible, as weekends are more costly. There are also procedures that do not occur on weekends which gives everyone, staff and patients, a break in the routine. The nursing staff did not have the time to run "herd" on Johnathan. Starting off on the wrong foot on a Saturday morning did not bode well for the entire day. Johnathan had not endeared himself to anyone on this Saturday morning. Plan or not, things were already not going Johnathan's way!

At a little after two, I called to check in again. I wanted to go for a run and so was not going to be available to a phone for about an hour. Johnathan was in front of the television with a bunch of the other patients. The nursing staff reported nothing to report other than, because the game was on, Johnathan could be trusted.

I called back in after my run. Now I was becoming the pain in the ass at the nursing desk. They didn't have time for my calls. The charge nurse asked if there wasn't someone I could call to get the report on the game *other* than Johnathan!

Her tone and curtness made me know I had stepped on too many toes. She told me emphatically that they would call me if there were any changes, and otherwise would I please bug out?

I made some dinner, read a book, and had just laid down for a short nap when the phone rang. It was about eight o'clock. Johnathan had gone to bed right after dinner with his comic books, a very unusual, way too civil activity for him. One of the swing shift nurses had gone in to check on him and found him sleeping and hard to arouse. His vitals were slightly low and he had seemed quite unhappy to have been awakened. I got up, got dressed for work, and left home. I knew he was going to get his way.

I arrived at the facility about nine forty-five, looked in on Johnathan, I shook his shoulder slightly to see if he would arouse when I called his name.

He opened one eye, looked at me and said, "Sue? Is that you?"

I replied, "Yes, Johnathan, it's me."

"You're early," he responded, closing his eyes. He had not looked up at the clock, he had not asked what time it was, he had never even opened his other eye.

I suggested to the charge nurse that we call in his parents. I really didn't know what to expect. There was nothing in my train-

107

ing or experience that would allow me to really accept that Johnathan was going to die, just like that. No preamble, no major change in vital signs or symptoms, no big deal. He was just going to watch his game, eat his dinner, go to bed and die, just as he had planned. It was too close to one of Johnathan's pranks for me to be alarmed, and yet there was just a speck of uneasiness that made me want his family there. Maybe he really was going to do a surprise birthday thing for his sister. Maybe there was going to be the best "Johnathan prank" of all because we were all going to be colluding in it. I just had no way of knowing what was up.

At ten forty, I walked down to the staff room for report. He'd already "gotten" me, because I'd put in two extra hours without pay. A new shift was coming on, my shift, except they had all had their extra nap or bath or time with their families. I'd been sitting there waiting for "Godot."

Five minutes into report, one of the nurses aides came running in to say that Johnathan's family was really worried by how he was breathing. This was also not unlike Johnathan. I pushed back my chair and headed for his room. Not fast. I walked at a normal walking pace, feeling a little bit like I was about to be had.

Johnathan was "cheyne stokes" breathing. This kind of breathing pattern is very common to an "end of life" episode. Stoke breathing is a series of shallow breaths followed by a cessation of breathing, and then as if the fire was stoked again, breathing resumes with a deep long breath. With each breathing series, the breath gets shallower and the intervals of non-breath get longer. I took Johnathan's vital signs. He was absolutely involved in his body shutting down. Either this kid was going to be up for an Emmy award, or this was the real thing.

Under normal circumstances in medicine, we would, at this juncture, jump into a crisis mode. We would begin to race around, ready to begin a life-saving process. The only problem was that Johnathan had made it very clear to all of us that this was his plan.

My emotions were beginning to ride a wave. I felt sick to my stomach. I turned to his parents to discuss what were we going to do. What did the family want us to do? We all knew what Johnathan wanted us to do. He had given us all our roles. He had defined the rules. He had dispensed with the rituals that were familiar to all of us. Now we were up to our necks in the discomfort of the moment. We did not know how to act out our parts in the final chapter of his life. He had asked us to act in a way we were totally untrained and unsocialized, to do.

Johnathan's mother and father began to tear up. They wanted us to stand by. They wanted us to honor their son's plan. I lifted Johnathan out of his bed and carried him to the rocking chair. He was so very light. I am not a very big person. I was no bigger in those years, yet to my one hundred ten pounds, he felt very light. I sat down holding him just as he had told me to do. I cradled him close and rocked. I could not whistle. I could not sing. I tried, but my voice cracked. The tears welled up in my eyes. I hummed. Johnathan's mom held his head. His nearly bald head. Johnathan's dad wiped all of our tears. He held his son's hand and wiped our tears, over and over again. Johnathan died at eleven-fifty-seven that night.

I sit here crying all over again as I write Johnathan's story. All these years later, I am touched just as deeply by this child and his family. I am grateful for the lessons Johnathan taught me. He began my long and lasting trip across the then barren plains of understanding death medically, socially, emotionally, physically, and spiritually. He led me to conferences taught by Elizabeth Kubler-Ross. He motivated me to build an extensive library on death and dying. Mostly, he taught me to honor the dying process as genuinely as I honor life. Johnathan taught me to never say no when invited to a birth or a death (as opposed to a funeral). It is these beginnings and endings that offer us life's greatest lessons.

It was Johnathan who taught me that there is not one way to die. There is not just one set of rules or one set of roles that is right. There are ways of knowing that death is close, even though I don't know what they are. I do know that Johnathan knew. It was my fault that I didn't ask him how he knew.

I am grateful for Johnathan's lessons. I hold them in my heart and soul far closer than I hold the memory of his pranks. He taught me how to keep my perspective with my own children. Pranks are pranks. Death is death. Sometimes, the boundaries between the two can get blurred. The real task in parenting is to provide and be held responsible for the education and safety that allows children to know when pranks can cause death. Yet, when children are the patients, they are the only ones who can know when they are ready to die.

I am grateful to Johnathan's parents for honoring their son's wishes and holding me accountable for what their son wanted me to do. I had never been taught to "stand by," as someone died, let alone sit, and rock, and hum. I had never been taught how to participate in a death, not by *doing*, but by *being*. I had never held life next to me as it softened away into death. I had never held a dead body that closely. I had never felt a soul take leave as a flame ceases to burn. These are lessons of life, not death.

The Art of Appreciation
Dorothy

I had met Dorothy many years before I would need to see her professionally. She was my age and a very high-profile businesswoman in the community. If there was an example of a woman who had never met a glass ceiling in the business world, she was the example . . . a very bright, high-energy person with wisdom and leadership skills built into one body. A person . . . a woman . . . of excellence. We had shared child activities, community service activities, and common horse interests over the years. We had mutual friends and often crossed paths at social gatherings. I enjoyed our visits each time they happened.

The call to my office was not made by Dorothy? or her doctor. I received a "Did you hear about what happened to Dorothy?" call from a mutual friend. Dorothy, in her mid-forties, had suffered a stroke. Cardiovascular accident (CVA) is what appeared on the referral letter. It was all very clinical. The MRI showed extensive lesions at three locations in her brain. Regardless of how it was written on paper, or how it was reported by friends, the results were devastating. Dorothy was paralyzed on her left side. Her left arm, her left leg, her left eye, the left side of her mouth, portions of her speech were affected because of changes in the muscles in her tongue. "This is what happens to old people," was a statement I heard over and over as people in the community tried to make sense of what had happened.

Only two generations ago, in the early nineteen-hundreds, people in their mid-forties were old. We have so quickly changed the longevity table that we forget. Or, perhaps, because we want to forget, we do not acknowledge how quickly this shift occurred. I am thankful for every day of my life. Had I been born in any pervious generation, I would have died at any number of life's intersections. I am alive because of modern medicine, antibiotics, obstetric surgical techniques, and early diagnostic capacities.

I met with Dorothy, her husband, and her doctor in the hospital. After lengthy discussions of options, we all decided that a short inpatient stay in an intensive rehabilitation unit associated with the medical school was the best first-line rehabilitation option. We also discussed the viability of her maintaining her positions at work and throughout the community on boards and commissions. I urged her to take an extended leave from everything, allowing her to focus full time, without distraction, on rehabilitation.

The windows of opportunity close very quickly in the human body after a central nervous system accident. Over the years, it has become obvious to me that if we are going to be able to recapture neuromuscular use and proprioceptive (where we are in space) patterns, we must work quickly and effectively. Often, patients are reluctant to make such drastic moves in their lives. Such a move forces them to see their limitations. Who would choose to see themselves in such a focused way? It also upsets the sense of self to lose so many facets of one's self image at once. There are many patients whose financial situation simply won't allow this drastic a change. I am so sorry that in our society we are ill-equipped to help people in these grave situations. This is where a form of national health insurance makes good sense.

Dorothy had the backing to focus full-time on rehab. She did! The same level of vision and strength that she had offered to her business, she offered to herself. Passive range of movement, constant evaluation of pain, relearning movement patterns by repetitiously moving body parts over and over again. Water exercises while being supported by people, and mechanical devices. Seven days a week, six to eight hours a day of focused rehabilitation. A true dedication to self.

I urged discussions of having an occupational therapist come in for a home assessment prior to her arriving home, so changes to facilitate access could be made. They lived in a beautiful home on a very steep hill, multiple levels and many stairs. Initially, we knew she would come home in a wheelchair. Some easy, user-friendly changes were made. I knew it was going to require a move in the long run. Neither Dorothy nor her husband was ready for the discussion. Part of their ability to keep moving forward was holding on to the hope that she would fully recover. Often a measure of denial is important to our survival. The trick is to keep denial in balance with reality.

Dorothy and the wheelchair never got along very well. It was a hate-hate relationship from the moment she sat down in it. She hated the seat, she hated the width, she kept hitting her hands as she went around corners. After watching her maneuver one day in the hall at the clinic, I realized she was not accurately judging distances well. Watching more closely, I noticed that she turned her head to the left each time she needed to maneuver a corner to the left. It was then that I realized she was using her right eye and her depth perception was being skewed. Back to the opthamologist. More work up, more exercises . . . this time with her eyes, more doctor appointments. Rehabilitation is a full-time job. To consider it anything less is not fair to either the patient or the family.

Dorothy's goal was to leave the wheelchair behind as soon as possible. Her husband came home one day to find her attempting to walk by herself in the hallway at home. Using the hall wall as the left side of her body, she would move forward with the right side and then wedge her left side along. It was a push-pull form of mobility. I had to admire her tenacity. We only went over the risk factor once. It was obviously time for braces and strengthening

113

programs. She was simply not going to take her rehabilitation sitting down.

Dorothy did not like the braces much better. She would look for something to do outside the range that the brace could move. Then she would go about thinking up ways to make it work. In one instance, this meant spending the whole afternoon on her rear end in the garden after she had gotten herself down, but couldn't get herself back up. At that juncture we all decided a cell phone in her pocket was a necessity. There are many times patients remind me of children. A new set of challenges to learn requires a huge amount of creativity. There is the knowledge, as there is with any parent, that you don't know what is going through their mind or body. There is no way of knowing how they are perceiving the challenge, and what adaptations are going to have to be made to keep them safe.

Dorothy was a challenge herself. She kept us all at work thinking of what she might want to try next. We had to be one step ahead of the safety issue. As her independence increased, additional and different modifications had to be made. She figured out how to sew elastic on the split back of permanently tied bow ties so that she could slip them over her head for a polished business look. There were modifications that meant wearing a stop watch around her neck so that she could see the time. With a cane in one hand, and an arm that didn't turn easily, wristwatches are tough.

The braces kept getting smaller as her strength increased. Her chief complaint continued to be fatigue, and the pain that resulted when the fatigue set in. Her fatigue set in each evening around dinner time. It is hard work when every aspect of movement has to be reorganized, thought through consciously, and adapted in some way. It takes a huge amount of extra energy to determine if perception signals are accurate or not. Is that really ice, or a shadow that looks like ice? Each perception requires having to go through a conscious process of thought. Is it cold enough to be icy, or is that a mental glitch of my eyes and brain? Everything takes more energy.

Most of us live much of our lives on the body's internal "autopilot." This is actually a portion of the brain called the reticular activating system. Our "knowing" is based predominantly on previous experiences or situations that the brain can "see" or organize as common or comparable to previous experiences.

We have all had the experience of driving home with our conscious mind on something else. When we arrive home, we realize that we remember nothing about the trip. We recall not seeing another car, a light, or a landmark, yet by some internal function we have arrived home safely. This is our reticular activating system at work, drumming up recall, under our immediate consciousness, from multiple areas of the brain. What a great inner-computer program. It goes awry if anything out of the ordinary happens, like moving into a new house six miles away. While driving home to our new house, where these patterns are not firmly set up in the brain, we may, without a thought, end up in our old driveway. Oops! Brain Spasm! Or, more accurately, not enough repetitious pattern for our brain to rely on, yet!

For patients with neurological diseases, or in Dorothy's case, a neurological accident, every experience has to be reprogrammed. That reprogramming also has to be redone many times as the body heals and strengthens. Each time the body changes, the response patterns also change, again and again.

We see this frequently in growth spurts in children. One day, they can throw a ball quite well and then a growth spurt happens. This is a window for neuromuscular reprogramming. When children are being rehabilitated, we welcome these windows of growth opportunities because the body and brain are expecting this reprogramming. Adult brains are not nearly this malleable. Perhaps, as medical research learns more about the adult brain, we will find a malleability enzyme or protein or neurotransmitter, that will allow us to turn on the adult human brain so that these periods of reprogramming can be done with more ease and less repetition.

Adults take safety signals for granted. Particularly, if they have had a negative experience doing something. If we have fallen off a narrow brick wall, usually we are considerably more cautious of narrow walls in general, if we will walk on them at all. In most adults, these negative experiences occurred when they were children, and the brain and body remember very well, and generalize these to future experiences. We count on this integrated sense of safety signals, daily. When we have had a disruption in our sensory signals, however, these safety signals are often disrupted. We have to adapt again to our external environment. We lose our auto-pilot until we can rebuild our database. This means each situation requires active mental participation in decision making in order to keep us safe. This is not only time- and energy-consuming, but often drives family members crazy. From their perspective, it should be living as usual. For the person reprogramming their neurological signals, it is all brand new.

Something as routine as taking a walk becomes a challenge. First, the person has to relearn the sequence of the walk. Then the terrain of the walk (for example, where the cracks and unevenness in a sidewalk are). Then how the lighting of the walk changes season to season and with weather patterns. The tempo of the walk may not be able to remain the same from one day to the next, even though the path of the walk remains the same. Frequently, it is easier to do the early rehab work on an indoor gym track where there is only one variable (the person) each day. The surfaces don't change, the light doesn't change, the terrain doesn't change, so if the person has changed that week, that is only thing that is new.

As the person's strength and coordination become more predictable, the environment can change and there can be successful adaptation. By limiting the variables in this way, patients have greater success and maintain their vitality for healing and growth.

Dorothy found that she simply could not adapt to all of the variables of their home. After several years of gallant attempts, she and her husband sold their home and moved into a condominium that had been built to be fully accessible according to the Americans with Disabilities Act's standards. In less than a week, much of Dorothy's nighttime fatigue lifted. With shelves that pulled out at working level, she had to lift a pot only two inches instead of two feet, life was easier. She was amazed at what a difference it made in their lives. She had loved to cook before her stroke, and now, with the ease of a kitchen designed to help her, not hinder her, she renewed her enthusiasm to cook. She worried that making things easier would stop her push to heal. Instead, it has had the opposite effect. She now has more energy to focus on the healing; energy that would have been used up in daily living.

One summer, she was able to help paint the exterior of their summer beachhouse by rigging up a paint roller that could be propped on her chest. She did admit that she propped it against her forehead now and again in order to hit the higher areas. This kind of innovation never ceases to amaze me. Clearly, humans are meant to adapt. Where there is a will, there is a way. Life's vitality will keep us survivors as long as we have the energy to keep living.

Each adaptation and modification lifts the bar of life a little higher. These changes give a patient an opportunity to see, feel, and acknowledge growth. It is important for family members and patients to take the time to reflect frequently on how far they've come. It is vital to take the pictures, laugh the laughs, appreciate and applaud the change.

All too often, we forget, because we *want* to forget, where we started in a process. It isn't fair to the people involved to forget. Often, I laugh while hearing the stories of the "weekend painting adventure" and respond by saying, "I remember when you couldn't even get out of bed, much less climb a ladder." This gives us an opportunity to appreciate. Appreciating, acknowledging and applauding are activities not done enough in rehabilitation. Even appreciating, while they are still alive, how people choose to die is important. Everyone needs to hear that we support and honor them. Every patient needs to hear how courageous we believe they are. We need to communicate and validate their willingness to teach us about life through their strength and courage.

Where Tenacity and Creativity Meet
Jane

Jane lived alone on a small piece of acreage outside of the city. She had a few sheep and two horses that she boarded at a large training barn during the winter months. She was a college professor, and a high-level competitive rider. Her competitive equestrian area was in a hunter/jumper class of riders. She was a very good rider, having won awards at many of the most respected horse shows in the United States.

All competitive sports have their risks. Athletes are most vulnerable in the early stages of learning and training, and at the later stages where the competitive pressures are highest. In equestrian sports, there are two athletes, the horse and the rider. In this sport, there is twice the number of possible unpredictable events as a result.

In Jane's case, it was a combination of wet turf, a horse that lost footing, and a jump with a combination of wood and cement as standard elements. When all was said and done, Jane fell off, the horse landed on her, she was on the edge of a cement footing, and her back was broken and her spinal cord severed. She was paralyzed from the middle of her back to her feet.

Jane woke up in the hospital ready to go home. This is a good example of good news/bad news in human behavior. On the good news side, she was optimistic and vital, on the bad news side, she was very unrealistic. Friends pitched in to do the work at home while Jane went to inpatient rehab. Jane moved on to a visit at home with an occupational therapist four months after her accident. When they were done, there was a plan for the modifications that would need to be made in order for Jane to go home.

While the modifications were underway, Jane went into a nursing home from which she could use public transportation to resume some of her work load at the local university. She found that she could accomplish her teaching obligations quite easily as her college was quite accessible. The accessability issues became foremost in her life. She had to make changes to her office. She paid students to come in to help her reorganize her "floor piles" to wheelchair-level piles on elevated surfaces.

She also began to get depressed. All of things that she could do, and all of the changes that could be made in helping her to live her life, made her acutely aware of all of the things she desperately wanted to do that were not going to be possible even with modifications. She hit an emotional bottom at a time when family and friends were experiencing hopefulness as she was back to work and seeming to adjust and adapt quite well. This created a lot of confusion for everyone. They felt they didn't understand her, and she felt unsupported and misunderstood. Not a good combination for anyone.

Depression is very real in people confronting major changes in their lives. Often it represents the true change in biochemistry that a sudden change in activity-level creates. Athletes are especially prone to depression going hand in hand with illness or injury because of these biochemical changes as well as major changes in self image and self definition. Jane was no exception to the rule.

Jane's depression had to be addressed. It became the overriding force of her life. Her vitality began to slip. Her interest in rehabilitation slipped completely. She began to reject meals in the nursing home, refusing to come to the dining room. She "forgot" appointments at the clinic and at the university. She "forgot" when she had classes scheduled, or would stop mid-sentence, mid-lecture and dismiss her class. She would misplace teaching notes. She failed to return phone calls or hand back papers. One student complained to the dean that her paper had been returned to her with an "A," but that every comment written on it was negative and disapproving. The dean was experienced enough to reassure the student that it was not about her, but rather a sad commentary on where Jane was emotionally . . . a painful admission, a painful reality.

Depression can be very elusive. Jane was not about to admit her depression. She felt everyone was being critical of her and demanding too much! From her perspective, no one could possibly understand how difficult her life was and how angry she was at having to make all of the changes she needed to make. She frankly hated her life now, and wasn't sure she wanted to go on living this way. All of the things that Jane felt were valid. There was still one very important question that needed to be addressed. Was there a biochemical change in her system that *required* her to see her cup empty, as opposed to seeing her cup as available to be filled?

Jane refused to take an anti-depressant. This position always poses a problem. A patient absolutely has the right to refuse treatment. In some cases, however, the refusing of treatment poses a risk to the patient. We all realized that Jane was approaching the risk of suicide. This is when professional judgment needs to step up to the plate. In Jane's case, a brother, the only family member available, and the dean of her department at the university, came forward to help with the intervention. Jane was re-hospitalized.

At this precarious juncture in treatment, a new doctor took over her psychiatric treatment. This is often criticized by the patients and their families as too many doctors. Why have an unfamiliar doctor added to the medical soup? The answer is two-fold. Firstly, a psychiatrist is by far the best professional to manage a depression and medication situation as complex as Jane's. Secondly, this leaves the primary and rehab professionals out of the first line of anger. They must remain as "good guys" in order to continue treatment and management of the case after the psychiatric intervention is completed. We all hope for good outcomes and stabilized mental health, so that rehabilitation and health can prevail.

Jane remained hospitalized for over a month while various medications were tried and therapy could occur. She improved steadily. She received daily inpatient physical therapy along with the mental health treatment. She was able to grade students' papers and supervise one independent project by telephone. Her university department chairperson helped at every juncture, bringing materials for her and reaffirming along the way that her position was awaiting her return. This kind of support and community care is part of what allows a patient to become vital once again. It also maintained Jane's health insurance. This is no small gift in today's society. The cost of medical care, and the availability of care without insurance, becomes a burden in and of itself for many patients and their families. Care sometimes simply can't be afforded.

Jane returned to the nursing home. On medications, she was able to resume teaching the following term. Six months later, she returned home. The sheep had all been sold, and her horses leased out at the training barn. It was going to be enough to deal with a new car, a lift, a motorized wheelchair, lifts in the bathroom, lifts in the bedroom, and new ramps everywhere.

Jane returned home with her friends taking turns staying with her for four weeks. Then, she was on her own. She remained in treatment once a week for several more months. In great part, this allowed us to trouble shoot the issues of interfacing mechanical devices and new skills of movement. Strength building at this stage is usually not a problem. Every task of moving oneself through daily activities requires so much strength that adding a strength-building program seems redundant. Jane's non-moving, non-feeling legs still required care and attention. Coming to the clinic allowed massage and another person's critical eye for injuries or changes in tissue that needed to be addressed.

One year after Jane had returned home, she bought more sheep. Everyone thought this was too much to handle, but Jane was relentless in her determination. She had paths to and from the pasture paved for her wheelchair. She had a pulley system placed in the barn for feeding and watering. She was determined.

Rounding the sheep up became the greatest problem. With the help of an organization that supports sheep ranching, she was informed about the use of sheep dogs. Jobs that she had done on foot before needed to have a solution; an adaptation. She "interviewed" trained and experienced dogs. One dog, an English sheep dog, decided at the end of her "interview" with Jane that she belonged to her. Shep became Jane's sheep legs. Shep also became a vital part of Jane's safety and companionship.

Years have now gone by. Shep's "replacement" is already being trained by Shep. Shep will be too old soon to do the work required. Jane still raises sheep, teaches, and now occasionally goes to horse shows to spectate. Her horses are sold and still being shown and enjoyed by other riders. Jane is alive and in life.

The Educational Power of Pain
Phil

Phil was a "fifty-something" corporate executive officer when we first met. He was an avid golfer. His lumbar back had begun to give him trouble. His internal medicine doctor had sent him to see a surgeon. The surgeon had referred him to me, as there was nothing surgery could correct about Phil's back. Phil's painful back was a result of inactivity—years of sitting and inactivity.

The human body is meant to move. We are not adapted to being in one position over long hours. We are not adapted to doing repetitive activity in a limited movement range over and over again. That, of course, is exactly what makes up most of each and every day for many Americans. Many of us need to *work out* because we no longer *work* in the true physical sense of the word. Just a few generations ago the work of everyday existence was so cardio-vascular and so varied in the activities that needed to be done, that we did not have to worry about fitness or even caloric intake. Our lives provided all the workout we needed, seven days a week. We didn't work out for thirty to sixty minutes, a few days a week. We worked out for ten or eleven hours a day.

Phil sat at a desk in a hip flexion, knee flexion, ankle flexion position hour after hour. Then he got up and went to play eighteen holes of golf riding a golf cart in between holes. He then returned to his desk for more hours. He sat in the same position to drive home, eat dinner, and watch TV. Only when he went to bed and stretched out did his position change. Sleep research shows us that when we spend multiple hours in a hip flexion, knee flexion position during the day, after only a few hours of sleep, we return to this familiar position by turning on our sides and replicating the position. It is as if our body and our muscles "know" this position so well that any other position feels uncomfortable.

Phil had to learn to stretch and change his hip flexion, knee flexion position with frequency. This meant changes in awareness and action throughout his work day, his leisure time activities, even his transportation. Phil was very responsive to these changes. He began riding the train to and from work, which required him to walk to the station. He focused on creating several work stations that allowed him to stand to do some of his work activities. He created a stretching area in his large office and had it equipped with a Yoga mat and mirror. He was determined to help himself and improve the condition of his back. A problem occurred. As his body changed, his golf game did also, for the worse.

For a golfer with an assigned numerical handicap to watch his game fall to ruins is a very difficult experience. He couldn't figure out what was happening. If he was feeling better, and getting better, why was his game getting worse? We began addressing this problem with some golf lessons with the club professional. He addressed the changes in Phil's stance and range of motion. Phil practiced, his game improved. Phil had to learn to play his golf game with a new body.

As Phil addressed his back pain, he realized that he was also addressing many other pieces of his life. He began to recognize how he was using his work and his golf to stay away from home. He also began to see how closely related to work his golf game was. Both "games" demanded continuous focus, competition, and very little physical activity. As he slowed down with stretching, walking to and from work, and carrying his golf clubs in between holes, he realized that maybe he had been going too fast long enough. He realized maybe it was time to really slow down. He was slightly overweight, carrying it around his middle, like so many middle-aged men. He didn't mind how he looked, because he looked like all of his friends.

Phil's back got better, but did not get well. He wanted to be out of pain and not have to worry about how he moved, or if he stretched, or if he exercised. He wanted more, yet felt like he had invested enough. He wanted me to "fix" him. I laughed and explained the next piece of work that needed to be done was losing the extra fifty pounds around his middle. I also explained that it was a simple equation of calories in and calories out. The calories out had to be more than the calories in. He wanted a pill that would take care of this part. I frankly didn't know of one that worked.

We tackled evaluating his diet in much the same way we had determined what had to be done for stretching and exercising. He didn't like this part of the plan. Where he had gladly made the changes on the exercise list, he did not like the idea of controlling what he ate at all. He hated vegetables. He loved meats. He didn't eat fruit. He loved fudgesicles and candy bars. He liked drinking. He hated water, and truly believed it would "rust his pipes." This task looked like a tough one.

I believe that we are designed to eat food. I don't believe in taking huge amounts of concentrated vitamins. I can't see where in human physiology we are adapted for their digestion. Vitamins are new on the human scene, and *only* in societies with huge amounts of disposable income. We may, in fact, adapt to concentrated vitamins, but adaptation of this sort takes thousands if not hundreds of thousands of years. Vitamins and minerals are well-balanced along with amino acids (proteins), fats and carbohydrates in most foods. It is how these vital resources are in combinations in our foods that allows food to work in our bodies. It might be easier to pop a pill than to eat, but I don't think that this creates health.

Phil and I sat down together and outlined a basic food plan

that included everything he liked, although sometimes in smaller quantities than six or eight fudgesicles each night, and a few things he didn't like. We settled on fruit or vegetable juices instead of cooked vegetables or fruits. The dietary changes began to work. Phil began to lose weight easily. He was very successful until a diet pill came on the market. Fen-Phen was the name of the pill from "dietary heaven."

Phil had learned that I expected him to come in and talk ideas over before he made decisions on health issues. I listened as he made his case for "just taking the pill." He thought it would speed up his weight loss, allow him to eat more of what he wanted (fudgesicles and steak) and less of what he didn't like (orange juice and vegetable juices). I listened while he presented his "air-tight" case. I then explained that while I thought his ideas were well thought out, I just hated my patients to be the guinea pigs of the medical community. I was willing to consider it, but not until the drug had been on the market for at least a year. I also suggested to him that he really didn't fit into the category of obesity that this drug had been designed to address. He left feeling disappointed that I didn't support his quick fix.

It wasn't long after our conversation that problems with Fen-Phen began to surface. Serious problems that were well enough reported in the general public by the media, that even Phil was humbled. He went willingly back to controlling his diet. As his weight came off, his back pain went away.

Phil was getting healthier all of the time. He felt great, looked wonderful, was proud of all of the changes he had made, and was getting ready to retire and begin to do the traveling he and his wife had always talked about doing. He was going to golf around the world. He was also willing to take a cruise that his wife had always wanted to take. He worried about the food and drink temptations. He was very excited when he realized upon returning home that without "starving himself to death," he had only gained three pounds in the four week cruise.

One year into his retirement, Phil had a heart attack. Upon being released from the hospital with more pills than he thought possible to swallow, he was angry, real angry. He felt betrayed. He felt I had betrayed him. How could he have been alive so long without any problems until he started "my" health regime? He felt his own body had betrayed him. How come as soon as he lost weight and ate well had his heart quit working? He was angry. Why had he worked so hard if it wasn't going to make any difference at all?

There are no guarantees in life. We are not in total control of our health. We can do everything "right" and still die suddenly. Without warning, we can still contract a pathogen that will kill us in forty-eight hours, even with all of our modern medicine. The illusion of control is just that, an illusion. In the midst of a health crisis we have three possible choices. Firstly, we can fully embrace what is going on and give it our best. Secondly, we can fall into a very human condition of denial. Thirdly, we can grapple with the ultimate question: *Do we have an illness, or does the illness have us?*

At this moment in Phil's life, the illness had him. He was unable to consider that he was probably alive precisely because of the changes he had made in his life. He was *healthier* because of the work he had been doing changing his eating habits and making his back healthier. Phil had to decide to take the next step and begin to exercise.

Recovery from a heart attack takes perseverance and will. Perseverance, as it takes leap of faith after leap of faith along with a steady dose of hard work. Will plays a huge part in both. The leap of faith requires that the patient believe that the exercise program won't kill him. The hard work demands that the patient will do exactly what is required, not more and certainly not less.

Phil wasn't sure that he wanted to do the exercise program before the heart attack. He was fighting the reality of the fragility of his body. He was not believing that his heart issues had not been caused by the changes he had made in his life. Was there any chance at all that Phil was going to embrace the fact that the only thing that was going to save his life, and the quality of life that he had just begun to enjoy, was an exercise program? Only Phil could answer this question. I, frankly, wasn't sure what his answer would be.

Phil met with his cardiologist and came away with information about the need for an exercise program and an exercise program. He did not come away with an incentive for either the leap of faith or a dose of perseverance. He began to gain weight, and thankfully, his back began to ache. Thank God for pain!

Most people laugh when I am thankful for pain. In Phil's case, a good dose of back pain was exactly what we needed for a great dose of motivation. Without motivation, in this case, familiar back pain, we could not count on the swift kick in the rear that was needed to propel Phil forward. Phil came in believing that he was having the beginning of a second heart attack. He was *so* relieved to find out that it was his old reliable combination of weight gain and back pain that he promptly began his exercise program.

Boredom is a factor in an exercise program for every non-exerciser. The athletes of the world, the born to walk, run, swim, or climb cardiovascular fitness lovers, are never hampered by boredom, unless they are slowed by injury or illness. Their problem is not to "go" at all, but to go slowly enough not to cause injury to themselves during a rehab program. This is not the case for the non-exerciser. Their preference is simply not to exercise at all given any excuse. Boredom is an excuse.

Phil hated boredom. Boredom would be his first, second, and third excuse to stop his program. I was a slow learner with Phil. It wasn't until we had revisited his back pain three times that I realized that I had to *use* his focus on detail. I had to design an exercise program that was so full of small changes and details, that he didn't have time for boredom. I also had to alter his program with enough frequency that he stayed interested. This required home-work on my part.

I had to learn everything about the cutting edge in post heart attack treadmill rehabilitation. Walking on a treadmill is so boring to me that I had not learned all there was to know about treadmills, post heart attack rehab on treadmills, or who used treadmills for heart training. I happened upon a treadmill program used for training FBI officers. The basis of the program was heart recovery time. This required a huge amount of attention to detail while exercising. It also required a huge amount of attention to the detail of keeping track of pulse rates during rest phases. It had multiple levels of detail involving speed and incline. It required keeping records of each day. Details of what was done, how it was done, how the body reacted physiologically, and how the person felt emotionally. This was a program made in heaven for a patient like Phil. He and I were about to learn a great deal together about "walking" on a treadmill.

Two years have now gone by. Phil has a level of heart health that his cardiologist still cannot believe could be achieved by some-one in his age group, who had never had this level of fitness previ-ously. Phil does not have to be nearly as careful about what he eats, as he is burning calories to assist his diet. Phil hasn't had any back pain since we launched on his treadmill program. Phil plays better golf than he has ever played. (Not being a golfer myself, this is by his standards, certainly not mine.)

Phil has motivated more exercisers and non-exercisers alike to be heart healthy than either his cardiologist or I. I suspect he has prevented heart attacks in many people who, like him, never knew they were in heart trouble. Thanks to Phil, they never will be.

A "Good" Pain in the Ass
Mable

Mable was a schoolteacher in her late fifties when she was referred into our clinic by her internal medicine doctor for shoulder pain. A full diagnostic work-up had been completed and nothing was found. Her doctor believed her descriptions of her limited shoulder range of motion and her reported pain. She complained that writing on the chalk board was so painful by the end of the day that she could barely move her arm by the time she arrived home. Night would offer her some relief, but the pain would grow again the next day. She was very afraid that the therapy would hurt.

One hour later, she could move her shoulder without pain. This was nothing short of miraculous, and seldom happens. Mable went home with three more appointments booked for the following three weeks.

The following morning, we arrived to a message on our answering service from Mable. We needed to cancel her next three appointments. She had gone home from our office and tripped and fell on her front porch, breaking her clavicle and humerus (upper arm) bones. She had been seen at the emergency room. Her arm was now in a cast and sling. Her doctor had told her it would be six to eight weeks before she could return for therapy and rehab. She also reported that she would not have to write on the chalk board very much during that time, as the breaks were on her dominant side.

Eight weeks later, nearly to the day, Mable returned for therapy. She was excited about having the pain relieved because her shoulder had been getting very fatigued "hauling the cast around." The therapy hurt a bit more this time as the arm and tissues were quite stiff from the cast. Mable was still very pleased and made four additional appointments for the following four weeks.

The next week Mable came in waving her arm and demonstrating how well her arm was healing with the exercises we had given her the week before. She showed excellent increases in range of motion, although she did complain slightly about pain and fatigue by the end of the day. The session went very well.

Again she felt immediate pain relief. She left looking forward to her appointment the following week.

The following week did not occur. One day before her appointment, again, the answering service reported a call from Mable canceling her appointments for the next several weeks as she had tripped over a cord in her home and fallen against a blunt object cutting her face severely. She had been seen in the emergency room the night before and had multiple sutures in her face. She ended the message by letting us know that as soon as she was released by her doctor she would call again to reschedule.

We did not wait to hear from her to call her doctor. We called her doctor. We were all concerned about the beginning of what looked to be a pattern. When Mable's pain decreased, her injury rate increased. We wanted more information.

Her doctor expressed the same concern. Three of us decided to meet, her doctor, myself, and one of my colleagues who would be providing some of the care. We agreed that we needed to come to an understanding with Mable of what was occurring from her perspective. We then would outline a treatment plan depending on what we learned.

Mable returned to the clinic several weeks later. I did not work on her shoulder, but instead began to massage her legs and low back, and talk about exercises for strengthening. She was confused by this. She thought perhaps I had forgotten where her pain was, and where she needed the help. I told her I did remember, but that since I did not want to cause her additional injuries I was not going to work on her shoulder anymore.

I then pointed out the pattern that we had noticed. She looked very despondent. I asked if she had any idea why she had been falling after her sessions. She said that she couldn't think of anything. I suggested changes in her balance or eyesight. She assured me that she had felt nothing different. She left feeling relaxed, but her shoulder still hurt and she needed to make sure that I knew I had not made her feel better, as I had before. She also did not fall or injure herself. She made it to the following appointment in one piece.

At that appointment, as I again worked on her legs, she told me that she had given a great deal of thought to my question. She could only think of one thing. On her way home from each of the previous sessions, she realized that with her pain gone, she would have to work harder at home. While exploring this interesting statement further, I learned a great deal about Mable.

Mable lived in a household consisting of her husband and three grown sons. She and her husband worked all day, but not any of the young adult males held a job. She would, upon arriving at home after teaching high school students all day, begin her evening by cleaning the house and doing the laundry that had accumulated throughout the day as her sons "lived it up." She then would go on to cooking dinner, serving her husband and sons, cleaning up, and then sitting down to do her "homework" of grading papers. Her husband and sons would watch TV and eat snacks. Often, she would not get to bed before midnight. Mable reported that when she was in pain, she could ask for help with cleanup after dinner. If she was not in pain she could not justify requesting help from her family.

I considered this a therapy issue and suggested that she make an appointment with a good family therapist. She would not or could not hear of doing such a thing. She informed me that in her generation of women, a tough woman just did what she needed to do. I began to resist her perspective. I then realized that, although it seemed like a tough position for me to swallow, it was her truth. I asked her permission to think of possible solutions, and asked that she do the same prior to our session the next week.

The appointment the following week happened again without incident. I thought that perhaps we had been making up the problem as several weeks had gone by without Mable "having a fall." I was astonished when Mable walked in sat down and told me she had a solution. She suggested that I could work on her shoulder provided she had another pain somewhere else. I had never considered teaching someone how to have pain, so I was a bit taken aback as to how to go about "inventing a pain."

Mable and I talked at length about how her shoulder pain really hampered her teaching. She liked her classroom and students, so a pain in the shoulder was not acceptable. Ideally, her pain would appear magically as she arrived home and would leave before she went to bed. I set about thinking up how I could teach her to have a verifiable pain, but one she could have full control over. I decided a pain in the rear end would be as good a symbol as we could get. Sciatica on command. Now, I only had to figure out how to accomplish it.

Mable and I began her planned sciatica by teaching the tightening of specific muscles. We wandered around her body practicing isolated tightening from neck to toe. Once she had the idea about specific tension down, we went to work on the isolation of the gluteal muscles in the butt. These are large muscles and can be easily taught to tighten on command. They are not easily fatigued, however, and to get a good ache going, we were going to have to fatigue the muscles enough to increase the buildup of lactic acid in the tissue, a normal by-product of fatigue.

We decided on positioning her foot to go along with the isolated muscle tension in her rear end. She went home practicing new exercises, not to stretch muscles but to tighten and shorten them. Exercises not to alleviate pain but to cause it. In all of my professional career, I had never aided and abetted a patient in creating a good "pain in the ass."

She came back the following week simply elated! She had accomplished the "mission" with only one exception. Her "pain in the ass" was extreme. She had done such a good job of turning her pain on, she couldn't get it turned off. We again practiced positions for shortening and lengthening the muscles and tightening and loosening the muscles. By the next week, Mable could leave school pain free and have accomplished a good sciatic pain by the time she arrived home. By taking a few minutes just before she went off to bed, she could reverse the pain-filled cycle. She was quite pleased, as during the week, everyone in her household had noticed her "gimpy limp" and had commented on how it looked like it hurt. She had even tested the waters and asked for help a couple of times just to see if she got a positive response.

The next week, we went back to working on her shoulder. At the end of the hour, she was pain free throughout her entire body. She also had the skills to get the help she needed. At her husband's insistence the following week she had gone to the doctor for her "hip pain." Her doctor had diagnosed it as sciatica. She had suggested he call us to determine if we should "work on it with therapy." When her doctor called, I admitted to the whole process. He was both shocked and delighted. He felt it was going to be a fine way to treat the problem and suggested some placebo anti-inflammatory medications might be just the pill for her to pop. We all laughed about the whole concept, but it was working for Mable. A most interesting adaptation.

Three years went by before we heard from Mable again. She was planning on retiring. One of her sons had married. His wife had also moved in, and was some help around the house. Her increasing terror was that her husband was also going to retire. She was not at all sure if she could tolerate everyone being at home. Her shoulder pain was non-existent. Her sciatic pain came and went on command. She felt more in command, so needed to command her pain with less frequency.

I raised the issue of family therapy again, suggesting that the issue of retirement could be utilized as the "reason" for seeking guidance. I suggested support groups in the area that offered "retirement" as a common bond. She said she was too threatened by the possibility of "spilling all of her beans" were she to enter any form of therapy. She requested that we do the same kind of creative thinking around this issue as we had around moving her pain. I laughed and replied that I couldn't think of a way to gracefully move her husband and sons around. We both laughed out loud at the shared image.

We spent a few more minutes visiting about getting her and her husband involved in community activities and using these activities as a way to set boundaries and define the time they would be together and apart. She left with the names of some therapists and support group contacts. I did not hold my breath about her putting those resources to active use in her family.

We did not hear from Mable again. Several months later, I read about her death in the local newspaper obituary column. She died of a heart attack. Adaptation can take many forms. Human will is little understood in medicine.

The Circle

As a child, I would spend hours looking at circles. I would look for them in clouds, pictures, words. I would draw circles, finger-paint them, make them out of clay. To my child's eye a circle was a perfect form. No beginnings, no endings, no special direction it had to go in order to be read. I could make one by starting at any point, and going in any direction.

As I aged, I found circles everywhere, inside the human body, outside as symbols of religion, philosophy, and humanity. I found circles to represent time and timelessness.

Stories are circles. We can make them big or small. We can add to them. We can have others add their part to the tale. We can repeat them over and over. Stories can change over time or remain the same. Oral history and written history are all stories. Stories have been used throughout history to teach and to inform. Stories have been used to pass information that is vital to the survival of humanity as well as for mere gossip, and for the fun of spinning a yarn or telling a tale.

These circles, these stories, have been about human circles. How we live and how we adapt in our living. How we die and how we adapt in the process of our dying. I have chosen only a few of the stories in which I have been honored to participate. I have bent and blended stories to offer privacy.

There is no beginning or ending in adaptation. Adaptation is the process of life through the full circle of it. We all adapt. We all do the best job of adapting that we can, moment by moment, day by day, year by year, lifetime by lifetime. As we learn the depth of the wisdom that is contained in our bodies, we will be able to celebrate our adaptations more fully. We will be able to hold ourselves and each other in honor. We will be able to laugh more fully and cry more completely.

The blessing is that we are competent as animals, as mammals, as humans in our ability to adapt, live, and die. We are a circle.

An Addendum: Continually Learning to Fly On
Sue

This is a journal piece written over a two week period while on a trip to Glacier, Yellowstone, and the Grand Teton National Parks with my son, Chris, and partner, John. It gives a day-to-day look at the adaptations and constant awareness that are required of us with illnesses, injuries, pain, and in aging.

As we got back to the business of driving on to Sandpoint, Idaho, I thought of the luxury of years of driving experience. Looking around, relying on my brain to sort the crest of the road, my body to respond proprioceptively to the "feel" of the car. These are changes I, too, will need to relearn. As my illness takes away my "practiced knowing," I will have to learn and relearn stage after stage of change in my body and brain.

On the morning walk at Grand Coulee, I encountered a rattlesnake. As I was walking along, the snake was snoozing in the early morning sunshine. We were both rather startled! He woke up and began his hiss. I woke up and began my slow stepping backward. He was good-sized, but perfectly blended into the basalt stone greys and shrubby overhang shadows. I thought as I watched him slither toward his stone crevasse how his pattern was supposed to make him stand out, sending an early alarm visually. Perhaps it was the weakening of the acuteness of my sight, or perhaps it was the luck of the early morning hour and its shadows, but there was no pattern of alarm for me. He slid away, all the while watching me.

139

I stood still watching him. I have always loved the movement of snakes. I had been taught for all of my childhood years to back up, keep talking, and be respectful.

In ancient times, when biochemical physiology was being set by the survival of the most apt to adapt, snakes, like humans were more often prey than predators. We will hold a wary eye, but given any chance we would both rather separate, in our encounter, than attack. Attacking takes such a lot of energy. For me, a snake is not an adequate meal to make it worth my while. For the snake, I am too large a meal for the energy expenditure to make sense. We both kept a wary eye. The snake watched me. I watched the snake. The snake safely in his crevasse would have allowed me passage. A troll-like bluster bluff: "No one passes this rock holding me without giving their knowledge of three. Give me warning. Move real slow. Show me respect. Then, I'll let you go!" My walking partner, again without years of experience in the three aspects of snake troll passage rules, was only willing to turn back—as quickly as possible.

On our drive east today, we encountered eagles and ospreys in nests. Some on the higher, platform posts that had been placed next to the electrical wires. Others continued to nest on the electrical posts, even though the "easier" platforms were directly beside the nests. It was as if they were willing to risk an electrical charge of death rather that spend the energy to relocate to the nesting platform next door. We humans are caught in this dilemma more often than we choose to acknowledge.

Tonight, at a ski resort, we look out from the top of a peak. High above a lake and river, high enough to look out across the foothill ranges of the Rockies, high enough to have clouds caught on the tops of trees slipping silently onto the roofs of the human buildings. The sun sets behind the mountain peak. The sunset that I am so familiar with as the final gesture of my day, is outside of my sight! How do I know it really sets? I only know tonight that the darkness comes.

How our location changes our "knowing" of our world. Just one week ago, in Nevada, I looked up to see a full moon and a trillion stars in a pitch black sky. This is not my sky. Or, at least, not my sky in my life as an adult. It was my sky as a child. Now, a week later, in Idaho, I have my sky of clouds and dampness, without the familiarity of the sunset ritual. I keep wondering how Indians of these areas "understood" their world. The limitations of their familiar time and space. I get to warp my time and space by car, plane, and train. I can go quickly in the same day, certainly in the same season.

Today, I bought gold earrings. An Indian dream catcher with three feathers. I asked the middle-aged Indian man what the three feathers symbolized. I had to choose between two different pairs of earrings, one with one feather, one with three. He looked at me and replied, "It doesn't symbolize anything anymore." Not to be out-played, I rallied back, "Well, what did it use to symbolize?" He smiled. His response was, "For men, each feather meant a totem or achievement, for a woman, each feather signifies the number of husbands she had." As if a husband was somehow a totem or achievement. I took the earrings with three feathers. Not for having three husbands, but rather for appreciating the male perspective.

I have had three important totems—my three "P's," as I thought about it as Chris drove. My *parenting* achievements. Those wonderful children who I have had the honor of living with, talking with, guiding, and teaching. My *professional* achievements. The skill and knowledge that have become the boundaries of how I have learned to participate in healing with others. My *passions*. Those activities and people in my life that make up the "stuff" of my soul. My three feathers. These feathers are the pull of gravity that balance my dream-catcher. My dream-catcher holds a small star in the center. The stars in my sky. The stars in my eyes. The stars that make up my heros and heroines. The stars that hold my center. My creativity. My monocular self. Indians do symbolism.

I took a hike on the paved roads after breakfast this morning. The TV captured Chris. *Why was TV important at Schweitzer mountain?* I wondered. Chris explained that it was in fact because of cable. These are the points that worry me about the future. I walked a couple of miles and decided that I could "do it." These days, I never know what I can and cannot do. Safety is important. "Because I can" becomes a relevant theme.

Upon realizing that I could in fact "do" a walk, I came back to the hotel room and packed for an adventure . . . water bottles, a long-sleeved shirt should the additional two thousand feet reduce the temperature to below my shiver level, something to eat (I chose almonds and granola bars), a camera, binoculars, sunglasses, sun screen. These are not great innovations. In fact, for years, my backpack sat in "ready to go" condition in my closet. Every weekend, and many weekday summer evenings, I left for a walk in the woods. This changed years ago. At the time I reasoned it was the requirement of time and energy needing to be devoted to children. Now, in retrospect, I was already ill and losing energy and physical acuity. My denial system was beginning to aid in my survival.

My walk today was balanced with my recognition that I had to give myself permission to fall short of my goal of the top. I asked questions at the shop where I registered about the easiest route. In my past, this would have been unheard of. The tougher the better; the longer the greater the challenge. I set off. The alpine creeks racing against the granite rock produced enough noise to fill my auditory senses. I found myself overwhelmed. I wanted to hear the quaking of the aspen. I longed to hear the sounds of birds and insects. I longed for the noises of the wilderness.

On the path, I passed another woman. I asked questions about the condition of the trail. I thought back to my father's constant conversations about how women should not be in the wilderness alone. His perspective was not one of protection, his tone was one of judgment. A *thou shall not.* I often wondered why it would never occur to him to warn my brother. It was I who had hours of training and years of experience to make good choices. My brother would have mixed hiking with beer. This mix was always against my best judgment and inner rules of the road.

The smells were all there, as they were in my memory. Cedar and pine mixed with juniper as I gained altitude. Overwhelming smells of wet earth and early growth. Flowers abounded. Trillium, lupin, larkspur, lady slipper, mountain rose, bear grass, monkey flower, stink cabbage all in profusion. Yellows and purples, whites and oranges all against a blue sky and granite grays.

As I climbed further up, I experienced the excitement and nausea of the high altitude. I've always welcomed these seemingly paradoxical feelings. I knew my body was changing. Changing in a moment, adapting in the here and now, not in a lifetime or over a week or month. Adaptation in this moment. I have always loved the physiology of altitude, especially in me. I am just very unsure of what these changes will do now. Could my muscles hold up? Would the changes in oxygen in my body cause too much spasm for me to continue? Would changes in bloodflow make me too dizzy to feel safe? I had no way of knowing. This is the part of my illness I hate. I get angry at myself, my body, my brain, my changes. Grace and patience I have never had in huge amounts. I get impatient with my need to have these considerations. Yet, I dare not consider ignoring these concerns. Halfway up, I realized I had not brought my cell phone. I laughed as I had vowed to myself to pack it. The games my mind plays with itself. *So there, brain! You can't make me totally responsible!*

I got back just fine and had a great walk, except that I hungered for someone to listen to my thoughts, speak their mind, create conversation around the images and feelings. I hunger for companionship. It is hard to find others who are willing to walk the miles both in actuality as well as in spirituality and emotional-

143

ity. Chris can watch *Titanic* and see and hear these very same thoughts and images but cannot tolerate them from his mother.

I then managed to get back to the motel just in time to pack up our rafting gear and head back up to glacier to raft again. I had a wonderful time on the river. We put in fifteen miles up from the west entrance of the park and rafted about ten river miles back to the pull out at the main entrance. The middle fork offers some good troughs and fast-moving fancy rapids. I was appointed lead paddler as I was the only one, other than the guide, with a large amount of white water experience. Chris actually has had a fair amount of experience, but just isn't quite big enough to paddle hard enough. I wasn't sure I could either, but I am always good for the try. I explained my situation to the guide, and we put one of the other men in the boat behind me in case I couldn't paddle hard enough. He didn't speak English, so I was to "demonstrate" what needed to be done, even if I didn't have the full power to do it. It turned out fine.

My skill and experience made up for the areas where my power wasn't all that it could be. Our only glitch was the breaking of the thwart I was sitting on mid-rapid on the third rapid, a level four of all things! This propelled the ten-year-old between me and his inexperienced father paddling lead on the non-rudder side nearly over the front of the raft. Horrified, I grabbed him and threw him into the bow. This momentum threw his father backward into Chris. It was nearly Chris who ended up out of the raft and into the rapid. Chris, the athlete, managed to maintain his balance. Other than where he took the elbow to his forehead, Chris was no worse for the wear and tear of it all. Staying in the raft without a seat for the remaining eight miles was a bit of a trick. The ten-year-old's mother wasn't about to let him sit up front from that point on, which was too bad, as it really is the best seat in the house. I assured her over and over that since we weren't going to be using the seat he really was totally safe. He actually would have been safer than mid-raft, where he could neither see nor feel the river. Oh well. What we do in our fears.

I adore white-water rafting, so was delighted to know that I could still do it. There is something about the excitation of it, the unexpectedness of it, the needing to be so in the moment to assess and react in advance of every beat. There is something so perfect about working hard in a drop and then being able to feel the let down and relaxation of the pool after the drop. There is such a feeling of accomplishment knowing that with skill and experience you are able to give the river your best shot. There is something delicious about knowing that you eked out safety in an unsafe situation.

I could never understand in all of my years of canoeing, rafting, boating in general why people drank alcohol before, during, or after the experience. I could never understand wanting to dull my senses to any aspect of the experience. I didn't want to miss any of it while under any form of anesthesia. Now, I have to learn to do what I do under my internal anesthesia. My sensory neurons just don't work. I wondered if I could have known that the thwart was going to break if I could feel with my tissue the way I have in the past. Were there early clues that I could or would have felt before this disease?

Had I been able to get any early clue, perhaps I could have spared us all that moment of terror as it looked like this ten-year-old was about to be launched from the raft. It could easily have been a tragedy. The raft most certainly would have gone right over the top of him. That alone could easily have injured him badly if not killed him. Living through a level four rapid as a non swimming, lightweight ten-year-old, even with the best life jacket in the world, would have been chancy. All turned out just fine in the end. I was glad I was there. I was glad that even if my touch sensation isn't what it should be, my reactive muscle capacity is still good. Now proven so. Thank goodness.

Today appeared sunny and hot. We decided on a hike. Returning to the Tetons, we hiked into a viewpoint overlooking Phelps lake. It was a fairly arduous hike up a relatively steep, rocky trail. Chris and I hiked ahead. Stopping often to view meadows (looking for moose), birds, rock out-cropping and wild flowers. John couldn't match our pace. I can never figure out if he is simply out of physical conditioning or if this is more a power and control issue. In any case, it is ongoing. I have a difficult time with it. I am attempting to push my physical capacity. To see what I can see, hear what I can hear, do what I can do *while* I am still capable of seeing, hearing, feeling, and doing. I do not have the energy to pull him along through my life right now. I am also unwilling to give up what is left of my life, with these limitations of my body to appease him. How are limitations interwoven and how do we respond to others' limitations while also responding to our own? These are such interesting questions.

After our walk, I decided I wanted to try horseback riding. A trail ride, or as we used to call it a "nose to butt ride," is about as safe as you can get. I haven't been on a horse for ten years, so I knew this would be an experience. Not to be left behind, Chris decided he'd join me. We found a stable that could fit us in, and off we went. Driving south seventeen miles brought us into a nice canyon along the Snake River. We arrived to the typical western sprawl stable, and I immediately felt sadness for the animals. Hot, tired, saddled up, tied up, fly bothered these poor animals had been hauling unfamiliar human animals around all day. They asked how much horse experience we had and I replied, "None." I didn't know what to expect of my body, and knew it wasn't the same body that had spent decades on horses. I mounted a bright-eyed Indian paint named Apache. Chris mounted a bay mare named Sand. He was placed right behind the guide. I was at the end. Dust. My favorite position on a trail ride.

At the last minute, one of the trainers, a high-school fresh-

146

man on a two-year-old decided to come along to work with this two-year-old on his way to becoming a trail horse. She was a good trainer, and was actually working with gaits and behavior, working him toward becoming a Western pleasure mount. This was her third summer as a wrangler and her first as a trainer. She really wanted to be showing and jumping at home in Colorado, but knew she could get good training supervision at this wrangler rancher, so in Wyoming she was.

We started out with great hills, great vistas, narrow trails, huge drop-offs, and wonderful views of the Snake and Hobach Rivers. Twenty minutes into the ride the trainer on the two-year-old asked me where I had been trained in my riding skills. I laughed and replied that it was along the same lines as where she had gotten her training. It kind of came along with the territory in which I grew up. We laughed about it. I however felt better. Obviously, what she saw in my riding and how I felt in my riding were very different experiences. I was already acutely aware of the lack of strength in my right leg. I was acutely aware of having to pay complete attention to the position of my pelvic bones on the saddle. I was having to pay attention to my heel and sternum positions. I couldn't just "feel" them proprioceptively any more.

I loved the vistas that could be achieved on horseback. We climbed up to the brim of the hillside to look down into river valleys, across at the steep, jagged cliffs of the Tetons. I delighted at the sights, sounds, and smells of being on horseback. I did not delight in the dust. I remembered being able to relax my body on a horse. To post against a rough trot, or merely rock my pelvis into a smooth gaited walk. I remember in my brain, but I find I don't have enough feedback in my body now to find the internal rhythm. I want it back. I felt the sadness well up inside me. I felt the warmth of the tears against my eyes. I dared not allow the tears as I was so dusty that my face would turn to mud. I wiped my eyes with my arm. My arm turned to mud.

I believe that if we need to cry, we will. We only have the choice of crying outside or inside. So many tears are called sore throats, allergies, or stuffy noses. I swallow my tears. I cannot swallow the sadness nor the loss. I wonder if I can ever really do this again. I want to ride, but I cannot know if I am really safe, or if I possess the energy for the concentration that it takes. I guess this is the sensation one has in aging. The memory of what you could do persists, but the strength or muscular integrity simply doesn't.

I am too young. That is my own internal conflict. I say this laughingly because it is my own words I immediately hear in my head, *We're not supposed to live this long. We will get better at it. We will adapt. It just won't be in your lifetime or mine.* These words I have spoken for years in pathophysiology and physiology classes. I now face the irony of self-recognition. I've never been very good at this part of life. Self-limitation has always been taken as a form of challenge. I take it on, like a race or a game. A game to win. Self against self-limitation. It is a blessing and burden, a good news, bad news paradox to come face to face with not being able to play. Reality faces down the competition.

Returning to the hotel, I went for a swim in the lap pool. Lap after lap, I swam, forty in all. Here, I can still find rhythm. Here I can still feel my body. The buoyancy pushes the edges of my lack of awareness back. Maybe it is because I have swum more miles than I have ridden. Maybe it is the return to water. Maybe it is truly being out of gravity to some extent. I can't tell. I do know that in the water I can feel my body differently. I tune in even more. What is it? I realize I can't *feel* the water on my skin like I used to. I can't *feel* my bathing suit clinging or rubbing against my skin. I cannot feel the changes in water splashing against my body as I turn, the way that I know in my mind's memory that I should feel. I can feel the pressure of my pushing off against the wall with my feet. I can discern my muscles, just not my skin. In a weird way it is fun to do these little internal experiments. I just wish I could type them up and put them away for the night and have my own body back at the end of the experience.

I used to love the glide of my swim stroke. I knew as a competitive swimmer that often I used the glide phase as a rest, losing my competitive edge in the moment. I'd have coaches yell at me that I had a lazy swimmer's habit in my glide. I relished it. I relished the feel of the water passing over my skin as I pushed away from the wall. I loved the sensation as the water swept from my fingertips to my toes, touching, caressing every inch of my body as it swept by. I felt the power of the water and therefore the power of my body. I think the joy of swimming came equally in power and challenge in the glide and in the breath. It was in these moments that I could perceive the grace and wonder of "beating" the water at its game of drowning me. To stay alive in an environment not suitable for humans. To race against its gravity to pull me to the bottom. To push and pull against each of its molecules in such a way that I stayed "up." Above its depths I could glide. I could move. I could master.

Gliding is as close to floating as it ever gets in competitive swimming. Nowadays, I play with floating. My body has enough fat to float on water. As a child and teenager I simply could not float. I could hold my breath a long time, so I was always the victim who could and would lie on the bottom of the pool for lifesaving class drills. At the time, it was a skill I took pride in. Now, I look back and realize that this too was just part of the game. I could even look like death in the water and still have it beat. What an odd competition I've played with the Earth. Perhaps this is the "joy" of my disease . . . that I can have an all-new experience of the Earth. I will have to experience it without the elements of competition and challenge. An altogether new challenge.

After dinner John and I went to hear the first performance at the Teton Music Festival, a great set of musical pieces exploring the change in styles for the organ and brass. A musical exploration from the sixteenth century to the present. A classical delight of sound. Now, I often need to close my eyes while I listen to concerts. I cannot do all of my senses at once at the end of the day. I can't concentrate hard enough to do multi-phasic, multi-sensory tasks. This is a change for a person who has been able to easily sort data on several tracks.

Night brought pain and gut spasms. Sometimes I think this is the "body" price I pay when I push too hard during the day. I still can't get a handle on this. Is it something I eat, is it how much I do? Is it the number of tears in that day I "swallow down" that ends up upsetting my body when I try to relax? This is another set of experiments that I need to conduct on myself. The hardest part of these experiments is having to find the control piece. Doing nothing at all to determine if my body reacts differently. I find neither reward nor comfort in sitting still.

At Craters of the Moon National Monument, we walked out on the paths through land so harsh it is hard to imagine either an Indian or covered wagon managing their way, yet both did. It is hard to believe that a bird or tree could grow, yet they do. Bees pollinate wild flowers. Birds build nests and find enough food for their young. Foxes den up in the caves left from gas bubbles millennia ago. They find themselves food; they find each other to breed and continue the species here among the flows. Trenches, rifts, valleys, caves, spires, evidence of molten lava left behind, long cooled, heavenly cool in the heat of the summer sun.

I enter the Indian cave. "It doesn't need artificial light," the visitors center ranger had informed me. The ranger had recommended long pants and boots. I had neither readily available. I climbed in anyway. The coolness hit me in the face. The air was cooler to breathe. I understood the Indians. The caves had been their refuge in the summer. The caves had been their refuge in the winter. The caves had been their source of safety, community, shelter, time for survival, time for reflection. I walked more deeply into the cave. The birds had built nests on the edges. Here, they had the benefit from warmth and coolness, light and dark, cavern and openness.

When my eyes adapted, I began to see the formations I was picking my way across. The floor of the cave wrinkled or combed into line after line of flat ridges. The roof sheared or smooth, colored by this lichen or that fungus, bird droppings or water marks. These will be the very downfall of the cave. As the lichen's acidic tentacles reach further and further into water-rich crevice, soil will come, and then plants and roots, and ultimately physics will over take the earthen architecture, and the roof will collapse. Will there still be humans to explore these depths when the nature of erosion eliminates the shelter of the cave? There are molten debris that look ever so much like coral. There are structures, crystalline formations, mathematical patterns that repeat themselves so often on this earth. I see convolutions of lava that could well be the convolutions of the human intestine; tubes with folds. On the outside larger folds, on the inside folds closer together with projections and porous openings. Here in the bowels of the earth, I find our own bowels' look-alike. How could this be? Why can I stand in dryness and find coral of the sea and human bowel the organ of our source of nutrient? How do these patterns re-emerge in such different places on our earth?

I emerge into the brightness of the sunlight. Now, I see human skin superimposed on the surface of the land. Human skin under a microscopic lens. Lines, fissures, cracks, crevasse, patterns of cells. The desert is hot. I am thirsty. The wind picks up my arms, pushes against my face. I stretch my arms out and run down the path, yelling back to Chris that I am gliding. This, of course, is a major embarrassment to the fourteen-year-old. There is no one there to see me but him. No one to smile in acknowledgment that even adults need to play, expand, experiment with the world around them in the moment. I laugh running behind him, mocking him, telling him I am flying in his draft. He begins to run, too, and in that instant, he abandons his struggle with being a teenager. It returns as he reaches an uplift and sees others coming up the path toward us. He stops. He demands I stop also. I don't. My arms still outstretched in the winds I brush by him as if I don't know him at all, thus protecting him from further embarrassing abuse. Further down the trail another teenager, apparently less distracted by my antics, asks if there are any caves ahead that he can go into without a flashlight. Still as a bird I respond, "Indian Cave." He thanks me and I fly on.